Art+Medicine Collaborative Practice

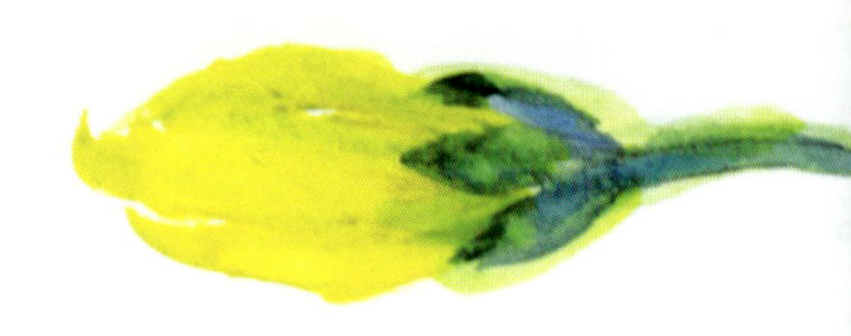

Art+ Medicine

Transforming the Experience of Head and Neck Cancer

Collaborative Practice

UNIVERSITY of ALBERTA PRESS

Pamela Brett-MacLean & Lianne McTavish, *Editors*

Published by

The University of Alberta Press
Ring House 2
Edmonton, Alberta, Canada T6G 2E1
www.uap.ualberta.ca

LIBRARY AND ARCHIVES CANADA
CATALOGUING IN PUBLICATION

Title: Art-medicine collaborative practice : transforming the experience of head and neck cancer / Pamela Brett-MacLean & Lianne McTavish, editors.
Names: Brett-MacLean, Pamela, editor. | McTavish, Lianne, 1967– editor.
Description: Includes bibliographical references.
Identifiers: Canadiana (print) 20190133015 | Canadiana (ebook) 20190133031 | ISBN 9781772124156 (softcover) | ISBN 9781772124781 (PDF)
Subjects: LCSH: Medicine and art. | LCSH: Cancer—Patients. | LCSH: Cancer—Treatment. | LCSH: Visual communication.
Classification: LCC N8223 .A78 2019 | DDC 704.9/4961—dc23

First edition, first printing, 2019.
First printed and bound in Canada by Friesens, Altona, Manitoba.
Copyediting and proofreading by Kay Rollans.

University of Alberta Press gratefully acknowledges the support received for its publishing program from the Government of Canada, the Canada Council for the Arts, and the Government of Alberta through the Alberta Media Fund.

Canada

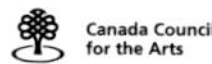

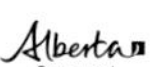

Title page: Ingrid Bachmann, one of four drawings, Untitled *(2016); 28.0 × 38.1 cm, gouache on paper.*

We extend our appreciation and thanks to all who made the FLUX: Responding to Head and Neck Cancer *exhibition, and this book, possible. This book is dedicated to all those who are committed to transforming the experience of head and neck cancer.*

The blurredness, indeterminacy of our sense impressions is not something which can be remedied, a blurredness to which a complete sharpness corresponds (or is opposed). Rather, this indeterminacy, ungraspability, this swimming of the sense impressions, is that which has been designated by the words "all is in flux."

—L. WITTGENSTEIN (1932–33), *Big Typescript*

Contents

MINN N. YOON

Foreword

The "see me, hear me, heal me" Project

> *Imagine not being able to recognize yourself in the mirror—see me. Nobody asked how it felt when I lost my voice—hear me. I will never be the same, even after dozens of surgeries and years of rehabilitation—heal me.*[1]

That afternoon, as I had done on countless previous visits to Starbucks, I ordered a tall Pike Place coffee. I was meeting Jane (not her real name) so I doubled my order. Jane had been recovering from head and neck cancer for over 10 years. As an assistant professor and researcher in the School of Dentistry at the University of Alberta, I was considering developing a qualitative study about the experience of being diagnosed with and treated for head and neck cancer. Jane had agreed to meet and share her experiences with me. As I waited, I was comforted by the familiar buzz of music, barista machines, and café chatter. I sat down and took a welcome sip of my coffee. The complex aroma of the warm brew heightened my sense of satisfaction and comfort.

Jane arrived. As we grew more comfortable with one another, Jane shared stories about how she came to learn that she had oropharyngeal cancer. She described the many treatments and surgeries she experienced after receiving her diagnosis and her continuing rehabilitation over the past decade. She relayed details regarding the extensive impact that head and neck cancer had wrought on all aspects of her life—physically, emotionally, and socially. As we prepared to leave, she shared with a rueful chuckle that she hoped one day she would be able to go through a coffee shop drive-through, have her order understood by the attendant, and actually be able to drink a coffee.

I looked at the coffee I had ordered for Jane two hours earlier. It sat on the table in front of her, untouched. All that I had not noticed during our time together began to overwhelm me. I was flooded by insights that, only in that moment, I truly began to understand. I realized that the ambient background noise of the coffee shop had impeded Jane's ability to communicate. As a result of the

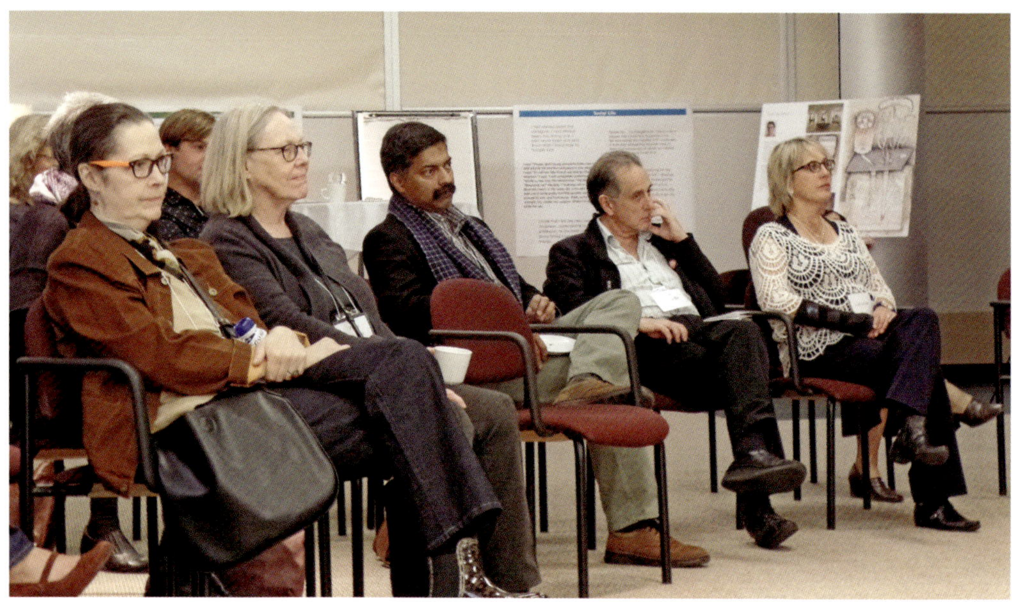

Initial workshop, "see me, hear me, heal me": Transforming Understandings of Patients' Experiences of Head and Neck Cancer, with David Diamond, Artistic Director, Theatre for Living (Vancouver, BC), seated second from the right.
October 30, 2015.
Photo: Nicole Schafenacker

surgical procedures she had undergone, she could not easily adjust the volume of her voice. The radiation therapy she had experienced had altered her sensory receptors. She could neither smell nor taste the coffee I had bought for her. The majority of her tongue base had been removed and replaced with tissue from her thigh, leaving her with a swallowing impairment that would cause her to choke if she drank thin liquids.

My meeting with Jane deeply touched me and marked the beginning of not only a new study, but also a new research path. I left our meeting compelled to help share the stories of those who have experienced head and neck cancer by making their complex, multilayered experiences visible to others through visual means as well as text.

Since 2015, as the lead of the "see me, hear me, heal me" project, I have had the privilege of exploring patients' experiences of head and neck cancer with an amazing group of artists, researchers, and health care providers at the University of Alberta. These include Pamela Brett-MacLean (Psychiatry; Arts & Humanities in Health & Medicine), Sean Caulfield (Art & Design), Lianne McTavish (Art & Design), Suresh Nayar (Surgery), Bradley Necyk (Art & Design; Psychiatry), Jana Rieger (Rehabilitation Medicine), and Helen Vallianatos (Anthropology).

Conceived as an interdisciplinary art–medicine project, "see me, hear me, heal me" (livingstories.ca/smhmhm) quickly expanded to include other eminent and emerging artists. Together we have been listening to, learning from, and collaborating with patients and

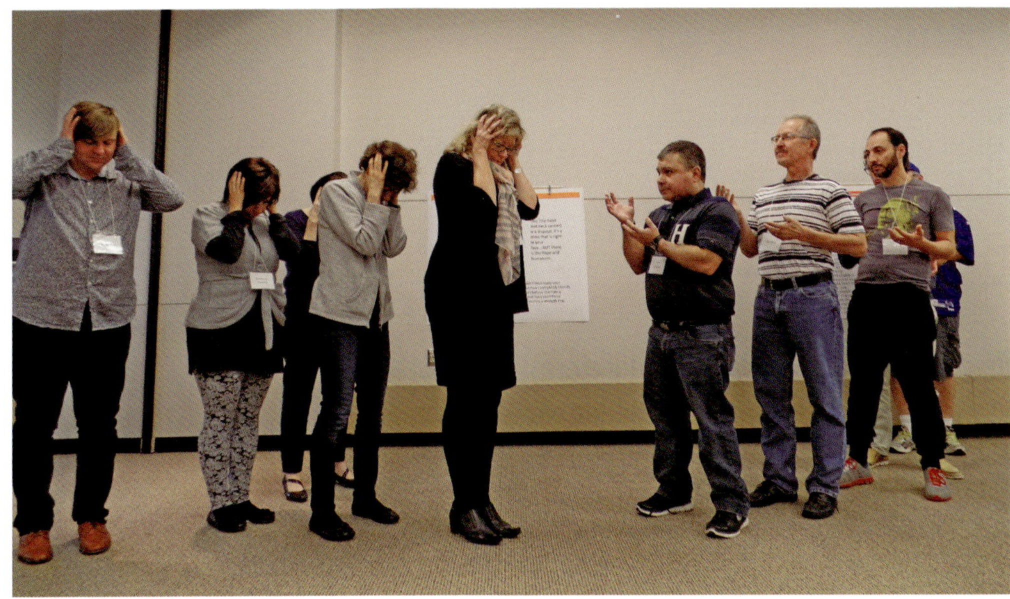

Initial workshop, "see me, hear me, heal me": Transforming Understandings of Patients' Experiences of Head and Neck Cancer, "frozen image" created and elaborated by patient and artist participants. October 30, 2015.
Photo: Nicole Schafenacker

family members impacted by head and neck cancer. Among the many patients and family members who participated in this project, I am pleased to recognize (with permission): Sharon Dixon, Kimberly Flowers, Deborah Hall-Lavoie, Eileen Kennedy, Bernie Krewski, Leslie O'Connor-Parsons, Ken Roth, Patricia Siferd, and M.L. Williamson.

We believe the "see me, hear me, heal me" project offers a model for transformative patient engagement in both health and arts-based research domains. Our collective journey has progressed through a series of meetings, workshops, interviews, and group studio visits, all of which helped build the scholarly and relational foundations for our project. An important beginning point can be traced to a workshop, held in October 2015, that brought patients and family members together with artists, health care providers, researchers, and representatives from Alberta Health Services and other health care agencies. Facilitated by David Diamond, Artistic Director, Theatre for Living (Vancouver, BC), the workshop engaged everyone in a participatory, theatre-based exploration of physical and verbal expressions of the pain, anxiety, and hope felt by those impacted by head and neck cancer. This embodied image-making process supported an evolving, dynamic inquiry into the experience of patients and their family members by fostering a supportive and safe environment for honest, respectful interactions and exchange. Additional meetings and workshops offered opportunities for exploring our vulnerabilities, which fostered the formation of authentic connections between patients, family members, artists, researchers, and scholars throughout the project.

Our collaboration on the "see me, hear me, heal me" project led to an exhibition—*FLUX: Responding to Head and Neck Cancer*, which ran through January 2017 at the dc3 Art Projects gallery in Edmonton, Alberta—and subsequently to further exhibitions as well as this publication. Our intention has been to facilitate a dialogue around the experiences of those impacted by head and neck cancer. We hope that this work will be a jumping-off point for innovative responses—transformative processes, products, services, and creative projects—geared toward supporting and promoting their health and well-being.

The "see me, hear me, heal me" project and resulting *FLUX* exhibition illustrate the potential of knowledge creation and translation at the intersection of arts-based research-creation, health research, and patient engagement. *FLUX* features the work of a distinct group of Canadian contemporary artists who have international reputations and longstanding commitment to interdisciplinary art–medicine research: Sean Caulfield (professor of fine arts at the University of Alberta); Ingrid Bachmann (associate professor of fine arts at Concordia University); Heather Huston and Jill Ho-You (both assistant professor of print media at the Alberta University of the Arts); along with professional artists Jude Griebel, based in Sundre, Alberta, and Leipzing, Germany, and Bradley Necyk based in Edmonton, Alberta. *FLUX* also features design work by Bahaa Harmouche and video documentation by Kyle Terrence.

A powerful exhibition, *FLUX* explores the painful transformations of those impacted by head and neck cancer in relation to issues of illness and bodies that are continually changing over the course of diagnosis and treatment. Drawing on her extensive experience working with artists and galleries, as well as her historical knowledge of the body and medicine, curator Lianne McTavish guided the process of exchange between patient partners and artists, as well as the selection and installation of the artwork included in this remarkable exhibition. Patient partners, integrally involved from the beginning, and who continued to communicate with artists and visit their studios during the art creation phase, also significantly contributed to the success of the exhibition by participating in panel presentations, conducting media interviews, and leading exhibition tours.

In these pages, you will find original visual content from the exhibition, along with essays written from a variety of perspectives, including fine arts, design, health research, clinical care, and patient experience. However you find your way to this book, it is important to note that you, the readers, are also important contributors, each of you bringing your own experiences and knowledge to the material. Some readers may be challenged by work that asks them to consider the transitory nature of their own bodies, rather than the aesthetic concerns of individual artists. For others, this may be your first contact with contemporary art, being drawn to the book by a personal connection to the subject matter—perhaps in relation to your own experiences with cancer as a patient, family member, friend, health care provider, or researcher.

We thank all the patient partners and family members who shared their intimate, personal experience of head and neck cancer, and entrusted their stories to us. Your stories form the heart of this project. It has been a privilege to witness their evolution over time.

We deeply appreciate and thank all who made the exhibitions of FLUX: *Responding to Head and Neck Cancer* so successful, and also thank those who made this book possible. Special thanks, as well, to Blaine Campbell (blainecampbell.com), Nicole Schafenacker, and Wojtek Gwiazda (wojtekgwiazda.com), as well as Bradley Necyk and Kyle Terrence, for their photographic contributions to this book. The larger project, exhibition, and book publication have been generously supported by the following organizations and funding bodies: dc3 Art Projects; the Killam Research Fund, Kule Institute for Advanced Studies, Faculty of Arts, Department of Art & Design, Faculty of Medicine & Dentistry, and School of Dentistry at the University of Alberta; and Alberta Innovates.

As we continue to grapple with the multiple, complex meanings portrayed in the artwork created for FLUX and the immense response to the inaugural and subsequent exhibitions that have been organized,[2] we have come to view FLUX not as the culminating end-point of the "see me, hear me, heal me" project, but rather as an opening to ongoing inquiry and dialogue. It is my hope that the FLUX exhibition and this text will engage you in gaining a deeper understanding of the impact head and neck cancer can have on the lives of those affected by it. It is my fervent hope that together we may work together to advance change in our society and communities in support of those affected by this form of cancer and also those impacted by other traumatic diseases and illnesses.

I offer the following comment, shared by a participant following the initial, introductory workshop we organized to launch the "see me, hear me, heal me" project[3] as one of many beginning points for reflection as you experience the content of this book:

> *I am in awe of this community. This is the promise and power of the work—of us, working together—of bringing our collective strengths—our collective willingness to look each other in the eye—to see me, to hear me, to heal me—to heal all of us.*

NOTES

1. In 2016, the University of Alberta nominated the "see me, hear me, heal me" project team for the Canadian Institutes for Health Research (CIHR) Gold Leaf Prize for Innovation: Patient Engagement. This statement, based on a collation of patient partner responses to the prompt "Imagine...," was included in the nomination package submitted to CIHR.
2. As of August 2018, close to 10,000 people have experienced artwork included in *FLUX*, which has received numerous positive reviews. Coverage of inaugural and subsequent exhibitions of *FLUX* has included: Holmes, B. (2017). See me, hear me, heal me. *The Lancet Oncology*, *18*(3), 296. http://dx.doi.org/10.1016/S1470-2045(17)30116-X; Pratt, A. (2017, February 8). Canadian artists take on cancer. *Canadian Art*. Retrieved from http://canadianart.ca/reviews/canadian-artists-take-cancer; Cummings, M. (2017, January 5). Head and neck cancer art exhibition unveils hidden experience. *Edmonton Journal*. Retrieved from http://edmontonjournal.com/news/local-news/head-and-neck-cancer-art-exhibition-unveils-hidden-experience; Hayes, S. (2017, January 10). Cancer patients make FLUX riveting: Art show started with interdisciplinary medical program. *St. Albert Gazette*. Retrieved from https://www.stalbertgazette.com/article/cancer-patients-make-flux-riveting-20170111; Hoyles, S. (2017, January 3). Art meets science: New FLUX exhibit explores life with cancer. *MetroNews*. Retrieved from http://www.metronews.ca/news/edmonton/2017/01/03/flux-new-exhibit-explores-life-with-cancer.html; Young, L. (2017, January 5). In your face: Innovative UAlberta-organized art exhibit on the most devastating form of cancer informs, moves, and heals. *Folio*. Retrieved from https://www.folio.ca/in-your-face.

   In addition, see the review of the exhibition of *FLUX* at the University of Alberta Hospital's McMullen Gallery: Boissonneault, S. (2017, July 13). An artistic representation of cancer. *Vue Weekly*. Retrieved from http://www.vueweekly.com/an-artistic-representation-of-cancer.

   Lianne McTavish has also published an article about the *FLUX* exhibition at the International Museum of Surgical Science (IMSS) in Chicago, Illinois: McTavish, L. (2019). *FLUX*: responding to head and neck cancer. *Canadian Medical Association Journal*, *191*(3), E80–E81. https://doi.org/10.1503/cmaj.180818.
3. We collected six pages of anonymous feedback from participating patients, family members, artists, health researchers, and representatives from Alberta Health Services and other health care agencies following our initial "see me, hear me, heal me": Introductory Workshop in October 2015. Comments covered a wide variety of topics, including new personal insights, ideas, and questions regarding the experience of head and neck cancer. In addition, a number of participants commented on how they experienced the workshop as both challenging and valuable. One participant shared: "This wasn't the easiest activity for me, but it felt genuine. I have even more confidence, not only for myself but for the greater community, that we truly seek to understand each other. What a rich experience to have in such a short timeframe. Mind blown."

LESLIE O'CONNOR-PARSONS

Preface

Before the Beginning... and Then

I wasn't sure what to expect when I was first invited to participate in the "see me, hear me, heal me" project. When I began to share my story, I found it difficult; adequately describing what I had experienced as a patient was emotionally challenging. It meant reliving all I had undergone during my treatment, which included surgery, radiation therapy, and chemotherapy over an extended period of time. Sharing my story was also physically difficult and frustrating due to the speech impairment I live with—for now, at least—as a result of treatment.

I was told that one of the objectives of the project was to bring understanding of the experience of head and neck cancer to people who have never had to live with it. "Oh," I said—but what I really thought was, "Good luck with that!" I recall stating that it was impossible for anyone who had not been through what I had been through to understand how I felt.

Then, in October 2015, I was invited to participate in an image theatre workshop with David Diamond, Artistic Director, Theatre for Living (Vancouver, BC). This initial workshop had been organized to bring everyone who was involved in the "see me, hear me, heal me" project together: artists, clinicians, researchers, and interested members of the community. Although it was intimidating at first, I recall being so impressed by the number and range of people who participated in the workshop. I was honoured to be counted among them. It was an extremely successful and inclusive event that left me feeling both hopeful and much less isolated.

The artists who participated in the workshop were invited to create work based on what we had experienced there together. Six months later, we all gathered again to learn about what they had come up with. Although the works were all at different stages of development, I found them to be very thoughtful and insightful.

Indeed, I have appreciated the artistry and care taken through all stages of the "see me, hear me, heal me" project that led to the FLUX exhibition. Although at the outset of the "see me, hear me, heal me" project I was doubtful about what could be accomplished, I'm sure, now, that my story can be shared.

"see me, hear me, heal me": Artists' Sharing Workshop, with preliminary work by Heather Huston displayed on screen. July 9, 2016.

Photo: Minn N. Yoon

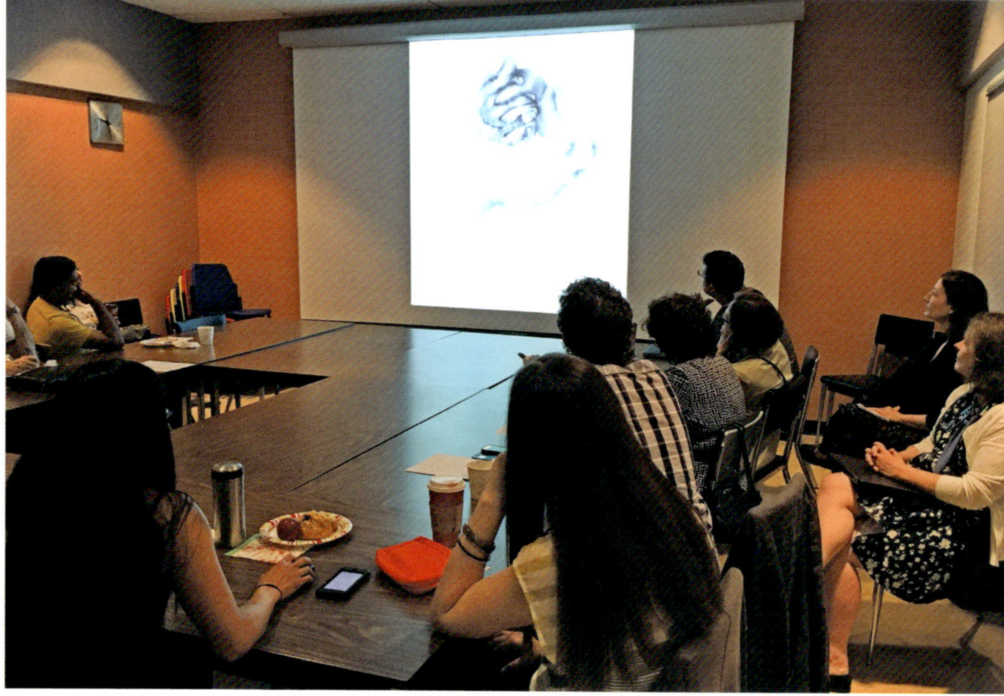

PAMELA BRETT-MACLEAN

Introduction
Expanding Relational Possibilities Through Collaborative Streams of Inquiry and Dialogue

And here we come on the difficulty of "all is in flux." Perhaps that is the place to start.

—L. WITTGENSTEIN (1980), *Culture and Value*

Increasing recognition of relational processes in health care has led to new directions for health research. As expert-based models open to more collaborative approaches, reconstruction of foundational understandings and purpose have inspired innovations in research practice. Relational processes that guided our collaborative art–medicine approach are evident in both the "see me, hear me, heal me" project and resulting *FLUX* exhibition.

With respect to these processes, patient engagement, which is vitally dependent on commitment to respectful, human-centred processes, combined with a focus on patient experience, represents an enormously promising approach to health research, offering a means for reimagining and supporting the emergence of a better future for health care. Artistic practices are also increasingly informing possibilities for research in and across disciplines.In a recent award-winning essay, noted social psychologist Kenneth Gergen outlined a provocative, new understanding of research, cogently reconceptualizing the purpose of research as "future forming." Such research aims not "to illuminate *what is*, but to create *what is to become*,"[1] by encouraging us to envision and work toward more promising future possibilities.

Given that what becomes knowable develops only as we explore beyond *what we know*, the question becomes: How do we create opportunities for developing insight and constructively engaging in dialogue beyond our own personal experience or field of expertise? In this context, we suggest the possibilities for developing new visions for a more relational, responsive health care system and world through processes of empathic reflexivity.

Awareness of fluid, always-developing "worlds of meaning" has led to expanding, participatory, open forms of inquiry and practice across a wide variety of domains.[2] Aligned with the heterogeneous, interdisciplinary movement referred to as the "affective turn,"[3] John Shotter emphasizes the crucial role of situated accounts in developing embodied, emotional experience. He encourages us to stop searching "for 'ideal realities hidden behind appearances'" and instead "focus on the unique concrete details of our living, dynamic, bodily involvements—or participations—in and with the world around us." Shotter points to the value of "unique-feeling-arousing" experiences that both serve to engage and orient one's attention, and encourage opening to new relational understandings that promote new ways of being in the world, thereby "enabling us to co-ordinate our actions in line with those of the others around us, and they with ours."[4]

A growing body of work at the nexus of arts, humanities, medicine, and science has emerged over the past 20 years or so, offering a means of making available a "kind of knowledge not available in other domains and inaccessible to other (more traditional) modes of enquiry."[5] Visual approaches have been noted to be "particularly suited to qualitative investigations of affectivity because the data already exceed the relatively narrow strictures of language."[6]

As a cultural form of practice, contemporary art aims to enhance receptiveness to and appreciation of the significance of the subject explored by engaging those interested in the outcomes of the inquiry "directly through the art itself."[7] In addition to the careful empirical approaches that are also employed by health researchers, artist-researchers use a distinct visual metaphoric or symbolic language to point to subtle, layered, often conflicting aspects of human experience. For both, insights are derived through all stages of the inquiry process—information gathering, analysis, reflection, experimentation, and synthesis. Within the realm of inquiry into the body and health, visual representations can offer conceptually rich accounts that provoke and heighten our sensitivity to subjective experience, as well as contextualize our understandings in relation to current and historical societal discourses. Contemporary art not only illuminates often-hidden aspects of experience, but can, through our affective response to the work, help to promote dialogue about opportunities for new starting points and fresh beginnings.

Hans-Georg Gadamer (1900–2002), among other philosophers, describes the power of art in relation to its ability to disrupt habitual expectations we hold, informed by our accepted "horizons of understanding."[8] He describes art in relation to its capacity to enhance subjective openness to others, and to other new understandings. Gadamer claims that "the work of art has its true being in the fact that it becomes an experience that changes the person who experiences it," which occurs through heightened awareness and attunement to that which is already in our midst and open to view. His description of understanding as a hermeneutical task emphasizes the importance of seeing connections, underscoring the importance of curation (or assemblage) in helping to guide how we relate to the subject of our inquiry. Our grasp of the meaning of interconnections between diverse fragments and components is significantly influenced by (and can depend on) how they are portrayed: "[W]e are certainly interested in the subject matter, but it acquires its life only from the light in which it is presented to us."

In his essay "From mirroring to world-making: Research as future forming," Gergen describes three promising developments in relation to research practices: 1) inquiry as incitement (increasing social consciousness); 2) research as creative construction (creating new practices); and 3) research as collaborative action.[9] The "see me, hear me, heal me" project has made significant inroads in achieving all of these aims. It offers a unique, collaborative model for arts-based inquiry into often hidden, highly complex, emotional aspects of a life-altering serious illness. Unsettling common assumptions regarding the roles and contributions of patient partners, the project also offers an exemplar for patient engagement. Our journey across life worlds and art–medicine disciplinary domains has involved multifaceted joint activities and complex processes of knowledge creation and discovery. Patients have been involved as partners and collaborators at each stage of the research process, even as other members of the project team have worked to understand and coordinate multiple, sometimes competing, discourses based on their own disciplinary positionings. The "see me, hear me, heal me" project has evolved through a progressive, relationally responsive process directed to fostering the development of reciprocal, mutually supportive relationships. Beginning with explicit affirmation of varying viewpoints and meaning frameworks held by those involved, we have endeavoured to support inquiry and reflection through information sharing, open communication, and collaborative action.

Further, visualization of embodied aspects of living with and through diagnosis and treatment has not only served to highlight and extend understanding of personal and social aspects of head and neck cancer, but has also worked to enhance "relational-action" potentials through the engagement of a wider public audience. The idea of including an exhibition of artistic works that would profile the everyday life and experiences of those affected by head and neck cancer, providing a platform for introducing new perspectives and broadening public dialogue, was experienced as daunting, yet compelling by all participants. Patient partners have shared that they accepted the invitation to participate in the "see me, hear me, heal me" project because they hoped it would promote awareness and improve the quality of life of those impacted by head and neck cancer. The artists involved in the project were intrigued by the opportunity to work directly with patients. Health researchers and health care providers viewed the prospect of participating in this complex, arts-based collaborative project as an exciting challenge and opportunity for extending their understanding of the potential of research inquiry.

Aimed at helping develop our sensitivities to, understandings of, and responsiveness to the impact of head and neck cancer on the lives of patients and their families, the FLUX: *Responding to Head and Neck Cancer* exhibition can be viewed as a dynamic sociocultural accomplishment. Challenging boundaries of separation and neatly derived, linguistically based research findings, the stark, challenging visual portrayals in the FLUX exhibition direct our attention to existential and affective aspects of the life-world experienced by head and neck cancer patients and their families, while offering a platform for dialogue within the larger community regarding next steps and new possibilities in the relational, social world.

The inaugural exhibition of FLUX at dc3 Art Projects (Edmonton, AB; January 2017) was very well-received. Subsequent presentations of artwork produced for FLUX have been organized at the McMullen Gallery, located in the University of Alberta Hospital (Edmonton, AB; June–August 2017), and the International Museum of Surgical Science (Chicago, IL; May–August 2018). Organized to help promote awareness of the exhibition, different activities and events such as opening receptions, curator presentations, exhibition tours led by patients, panel discussions, dialogue events, and film screenings have also offered unique opportunities for making meaning of the artwork. Each interactive engagement has offered, and continues to offer, openings to a relational confluence and a myriad of beginning points for discerning new connections and emergent new practices we may introduce in the world around us, as we work together in building a more promising future for us all.

The "see me, hear me, heal me" project has aimed to reach beyond a purely cognitive understanding of what it means to be human by encouraging responsiveness and the development of relational know-how to create new ways of being and becoming. Artworks created for the FLUX exhibition have provided a means for widening the circle of engagement within the public sphere, as well as furthering collaborative inquiry into the experience of those affected by head and neck cancer. We hope that this will broaden the range of possible supportive responses, including alignment with those affected by head and neck cancer. This project points to all that can be achieved by working together across divides in understanding that so often unsettle our attempts to build more promising futures for the world. Within the domain of research-creation and health research, the "see me, hear me, heal me" project provides an innovative model not only for patient engagement, but also for humanizing research.[10]

NOTES

1. Gergen, K.J. (2015). From mirroring to world-making: Research as future forming. *Journal for the Theory of Social Behaviour*, 45(3), 287–310. https://doi.org/10.1111/jtsb.12075. (Emphasis in original.)
2. Shotter, J. (2015). On "relational things": A new realm of inquiry. In R. Garud, B. Simpson, A. Langley & H. Tsoukas (Eds.), *The emergence of novelty in organizations* (pp. 56–79). Oxford: Oxford University Press.
3. Clough, P.T. & Halley, J. (Eds.). (2007). *The affective turn: Theorizing the social*. Durham, NC: Duke University Press.
4. Shotter, J. (2016, May). *Portraying "lived experiences" in "narrative accounts" that not only challenge prevailing "thought styles" in one's "social community," but provide enticing openings to change them.* Paper presented at the 11th Organization Studies Summer Workshop on Spirituality, Symbolism, and Storytelling, Mykonos, Greece. Retrieved from https://studylib.net/doc/7229231/portraying-lived-experiences%C3%BC-in-narrative-accounts.
5. Pakes, A. (2004). Art as action or art as object? The embodiment of knowledge in practice as research. *Working Papers in Art and Design*, 3. Retrieved from https://pure.roehampton.ac.uk/portal/en/publications/art-as-action-or-art-as-object(60f3db80-9828-49cc-83aa-a07ae9c841ee)/export.html.
6. Cromby, J. (2012). The affective turn and qualitative health research. *International Journal of Work Organisation and Emotion*, 5(2),145–58. https://doi.org/10.1504/IJWOE.2012.049518.
7. Social Sciences and Humanities Research Ethics Special Working Committee (SSHWC): A working committee of the Interagency Advisory Panel on Research Ethics (PRE). (2008). *Research involving creative practices: A chapter for inclusion in the Tri-Council Policy Statement TCPS—Ethical Conduct for Research Involving Humans.* Retrieved from http://www.pre.ethics.gc.ca/eng/archives/policy-politique/reports-rapports/ricp-ripc.
8. Gadamer, H-G. (1989). *Truth and method* (J. Weinsheimer and D.G. Marshall, Trans.). London: Bloomsbury.
9. Gergen (2015).
10. We have outlined our aesthetic, relational research approach in Yoon, M.N., & Brett-MacLean, P. (in press). Living stories: An arts-based, relational research framework directed to transformative change in healthcare. In D. Dole, E. Raboin, P. Thomas, et al. (Eds.), *Social Construction in Action: The Taos Institute's Silver Jubilee*. Chagrin Falls, OH: Taos Institute Publications.

In FLUX

LIANNE MCTAVISH

FLUX A Curatorial Introduction

View of main FLUX *exhibition area featuring the work of Heather Huston and Bradley Necyk at dc3 Art Projects, Edmonton, AB.* *Photo: Blaine Campbell*

Flux is a strong word that does not roll easily off the tongue. Pronouncing it takes effort. First the front teeth touch the bottom lip while the lungs expel air; then the tongue reaches up to the roof of the mouth, forming an "el" while the vocal chords engage. The jaw immediately lowers to help the voice shape the next sound, then closes again so that the tongue can press against the teeth to create a final hiss. This complex sequence of facial movements, controlled breathing, and use of the throat can be difficult, if not impossible, for someone recovering from head and neck cancer, particularly when they have undergone multiple surgeries to remove tumours, bones, and tissue.

As a concept, flux is nevertheless useful for thinking about the challenges of head and neck cancer, for the term has multiple, contradictory meanings. In contemporary English, it refers to fluidity and unrest. When we say that something is "in constant flux," we imply that it is both unknowable and unmanageable, attributes that can be seductive but also evoke fear. The word *flux* has increasingly negative associations within a medical context, where it

Printed excerpts of patient narratives in the FLUX exhibition entryway at dc3 Art Projects, Edmonton, AB.
Photo: Bradley Necyk

describes an excessive discharge of fluid from the body. The modern impulse to arrest this flow and protect the boundaries of the body is at odds with earlier medical approaches, notably those from the early modern period in Europe (1350–1750). At that time, the body was understood to be composed of four humours, or fluids, that were in continual motion. *Flux* was a term used by everyday people and especially women to describe the painful slowing of the normally fluid body. Fluxes were thus oppressive and burdensome sensations indicating an unseen illness within the body, a "stoppage" that was in need of expulsion or release. Despite this change in meaning, there is a central commonality in the past and present understandings of flux as an embodied condition: a flux is an unpleasant experience that consistently indicates that danger might be lurking beneath the skin.

There are also positive associations with the term *flux*. In metallurgy, a flux is a substance used to refine metals. When added to an impure metal, a flux combines with the impurities to form a molten mixture that can be removed. This sense of cooperation as well as cleansing continues in another, more chemical use of the word *flux* to name an ingredient added to dental porcelain because its low melting temperature helps to bond silica particles. These technical understandings of flux bring to mind the practical interventions used by health care professionals to treat head and neck cancer

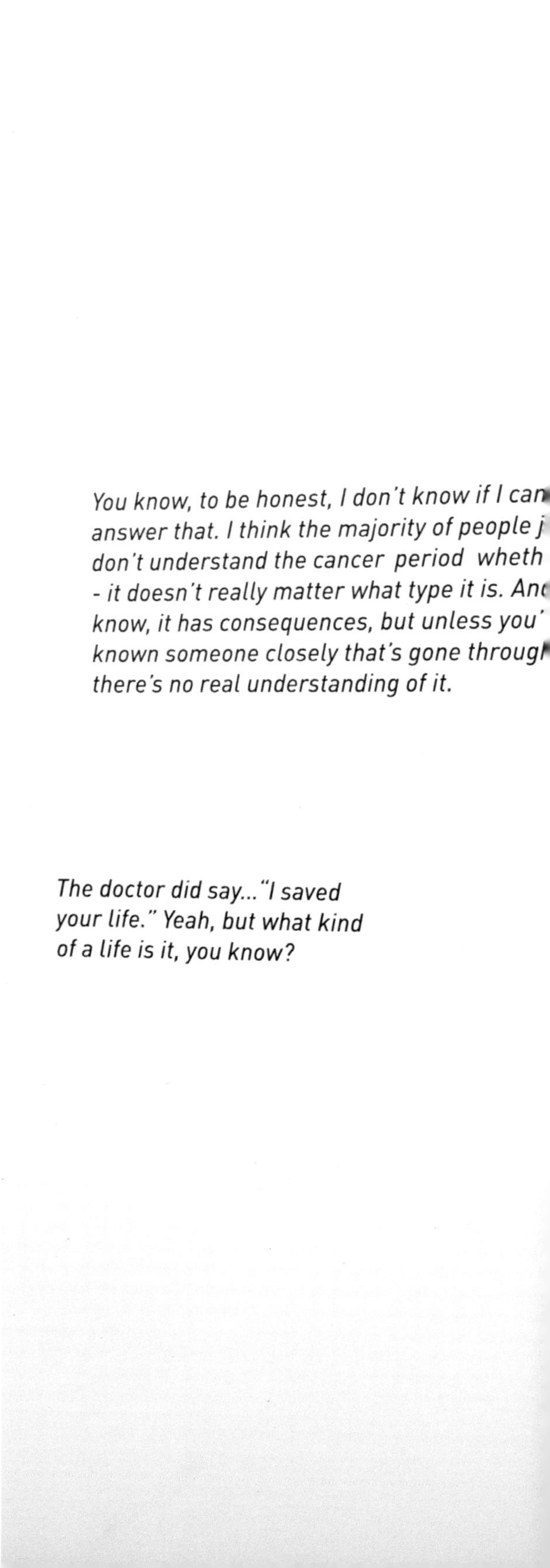

I think that I felt like I was surrendering my power...surrendering to the medical profes[sion] to the medicines, to society, to my family. I surrendered my home, my friends...

The first time hearing my voice...I didn't recognize my voice. I miss my old voice. I do get sad about it. I'm still finding ways to say good-bye to it because I know it not coming back.

The waiting is probably the toughest.

I don't actually make a sound when I laugh. It's just like a breath type thing. Yeah, and crying even. It's silent; laughing and crying are silent.

[...] a believer that the body is [pr]etty remarkable and it [wa]nts to, wherever possible, [re]program itself to do [dif]ferent things.

I made it very clear with my friends and family I want absolutely no photos. I want the mirror covered in the room. I don't want to actually see my damaged self. Part of that is admittedly vanity but the other part of that was also for me because I do meditate and visualize; it was critical for me to only have a picture in my mind of my healed self to focus on so I could get through my healing.

Well, it changes from t[...] perspective - your spe[...] changes. Your eating c[...] Your - what doesn't ch[...]

patients, including the careful reconstruction of the teeth of people recovering from invasive surgery and the effects of radiation therapy. Like a health care provider, a chemical flux participates in a process and promotes transformation; it is an active agent of change, introduced from the outside to encourage melting and reconfiguration. As an additive, a flux enters and then departs, leaving a lasting impression, much like the broad range of assistants—maxillofacial and dental surgeons, nurses, radiation therapists, speech therapists, and psychiatrists, among others—who alter, interpret, and strive to improve the bodily experiences of people with cancer.

While the FLUX exhibition embraces all of these possible significations, it highlights the ways in which contemporary artists, too, can enter the realm of head and neck cancer, inviting exploration of its meaning. The six participating artists were invited to collaborate with, learn from, and expand understanding of the experience of head and neck cancer, from the perspectives of both those who have been diagnosed with this form of cancer and their family members. By exchanging ideas with head and neck cancer patients, listening to their stories, and attending interactive workshops, the artists agreed to face the daunting and perhaps impossible task of representing the knowledge and experience of another. This approach was risky, necessitating a swerve away from—or flux within—standard methods of artistic practice.

Within the art world, this embrace of flux recalls the Fluxus movement, which developed during the 1960s and 1970s as an international, interdisciplinary collaboration of artists, poets, composers, and designers eager to produce syntheses of different artistic media and disciplines, and especially pursuing increased interaction between art and audience. Although the artists in FLUX similarly engaged in an experimental, audience-oriented process, they reached well beyond the art world to interact with people recovering from cancer and health care professionals, grappling with the emotional and physical outcomes of disease that usually remain hidden. The artworks that resulted from the collaborative encounters between artistic, medical, and everyday domains do much more than celebrate heroic cancer survivors. They convey the pain, confusion, catastrophe, and hope associated with a serious illness, showing that healing is an uneven and ongoing process that is *part of* someone's life, not something to be accomplished and set aside before getting back to "normal" living.

Jude Griebel's *Obstructed* (2016) features a steadfast figure resting on a bed, legs bent. This life-sized, gray creature is grotesque, a mountain hewn from rock and covered in trees. His monstrous face expresses pain; his spindly arms and legs fail to function. The path of these limb-highways is blocked by a landslide just below the neck. Transport trucks come to a standstill while other vehicles turn back. In this work, the body is a transportation system that has broken down. No longer whole, the body's identity is crumbling away—but all is not yet lost, for the ghostly white bed on which the figure sits suggests domesticity, convalescence, and care. This staging also refers to hospitalization because the figure is theatrically on display, offering up his condition to the viewer. Playing the role of patient, he is objectified by the scrutiny of the observer, who is asked to consider every detail, every decision made by the artist. The figure submits to this process; in between illness and cure, he is waiting for something to be done. All the same, the bulky form remains alert and strong, with energy kept in reserve. Like a god on Mount Olympus, his head is in the clouds. He is not, however, a magnificent being who hovers above and judges humanity. His body is inseparable from the natural world, both part of the environment and vulnerable to natural disasters. Mountains might seem to be stable, but they are always shifting and unpredictable. Sometimes they collapse, burying everything beneath them.

Jill Ho-You's *Veils* (2016) references medical treatment and the time-consuming process of healing after a traumatic event in a markedly different format. White mylar panels are suspended so as to enhance the shadows cast on the wall behind them, highlighting their material presence. Despite their rigidity, the rectangular sheets appear to be delicate because tiny sections have been meticulously removed from them. The resulting stencils are beautiful and abstract, resembling lace. At the same time, organic forms suggesting jaws, tibia, and other bones emerge from the play between positive and negative space. Viewers must pause and look carefully to reconstruct these bodily fragments, echoing the work done by the artist as well as the surgeons who inspired her choice of materials and approach. Ho-You developed her method of creation after visiting the Institute for Reconstructive Sciences in Medicine (IRSM) at the Misericordia Hospital in Edmonton, Alberta, to learn how specialists operate on people with head and neck cancer. Subsequently receiving a series of bone scans from the dental surgeons, she refabricated the images in mylar, a material that, like flesh, is both resistant and precarious. The artist used sharp razor blades and intense physical effort to cut patterned shapes from the panels. This process required her full attention because mylar, though tough, creases easily, leaving a scar that can never be erased. The final result hovers between the medical and aesthetic realms to mark their interdependence, providing evocative layers of meaning for the viewer to discover.

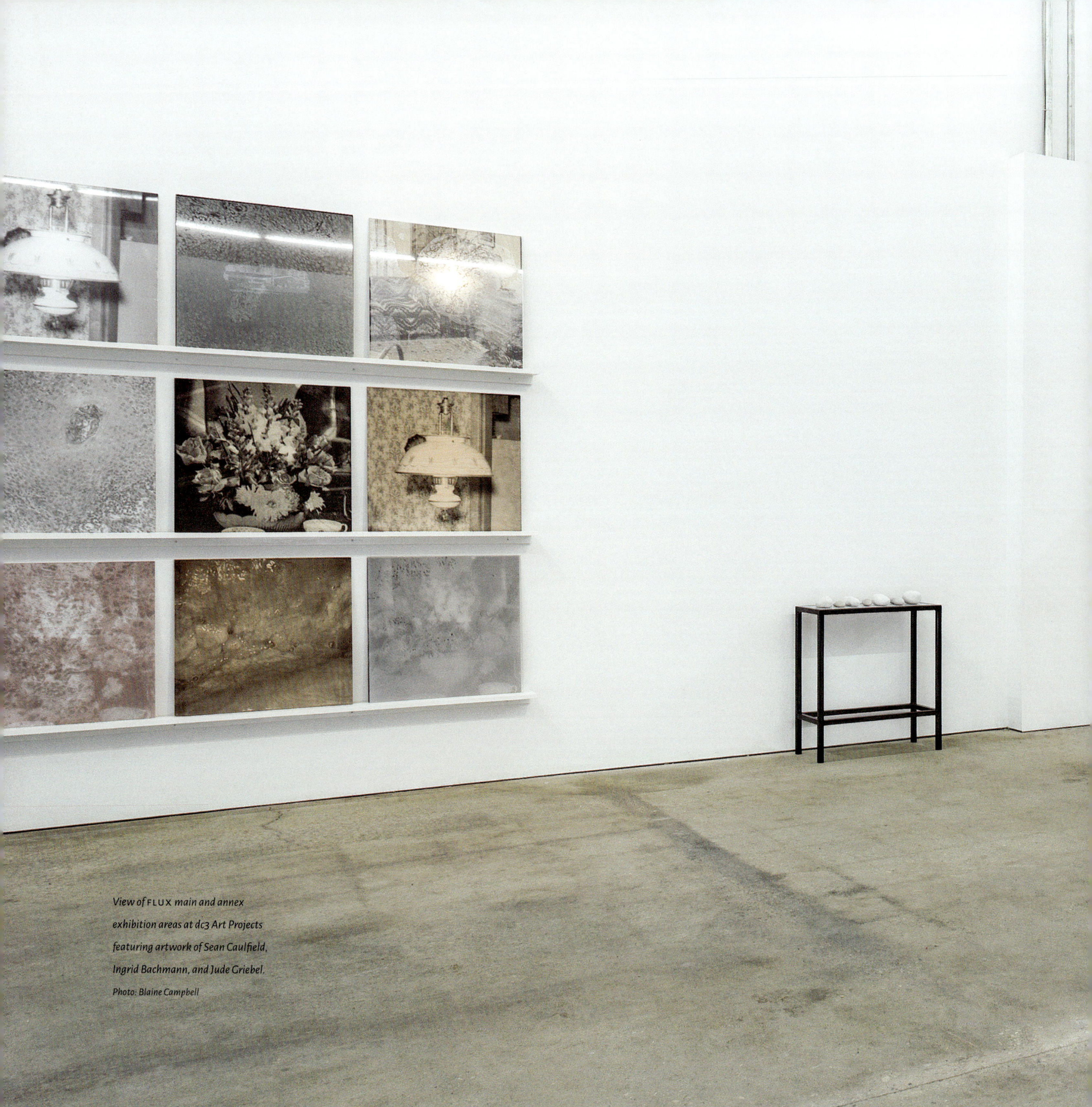

View of FLUX *main and annex exhibition areas at dc3 Art Projects featuring artwork of Sean Caulfield, Ingrid Bachmann, and Jude Griebel.*
Photo: Blaine Campbell

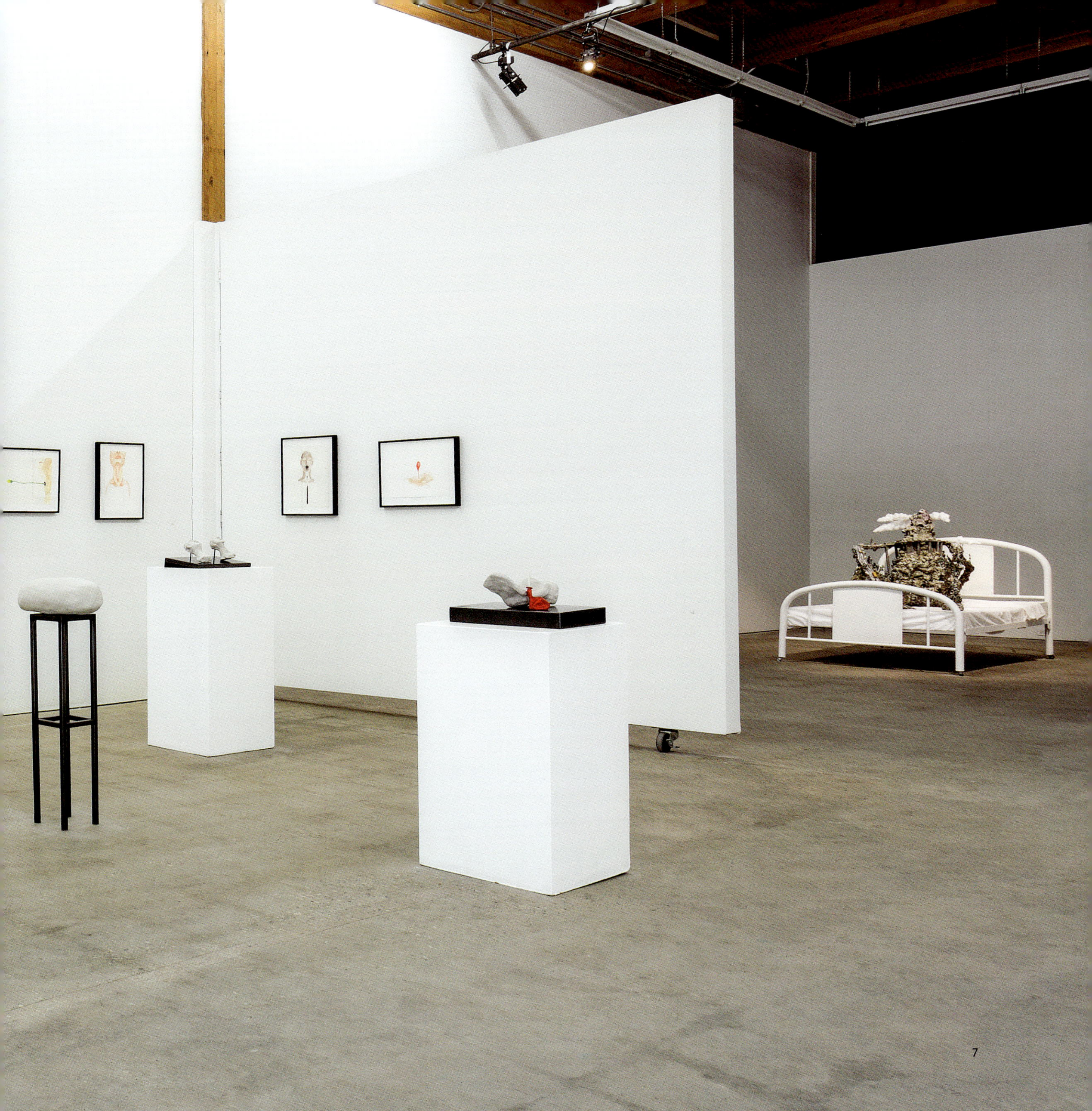

Ingrid Bachmann created a series of works inspired by her poetic responses to the stories of people recovering from cancer, including clay figures, gouache drawings, and a sound piece. A modelled clay throat and lower jaw rest on a base, offering visual access. Imprints of the artist's active hands indicate that the bodily fragment is an expressive medium, not an anatomical specimen. Signs of life return in a small red balloon that slowly expands and deflates by means of a tube inserted in an opening in the throat. The hole resembles a laryngectomy scar, the result of an invasive surgery that ensures survival while damaging the ability to swallow, speak, and eat. Although balloons are typically associated with celebration, this one fills with fluid rather than air, becoming strangely awkward. Two smaller clay heads are raised on a diagonal plinth, as if reclining in a dental chair. With roughly formed features and open mouths, the figures are clearly human but are not individualized portrait busts. A small hole pierces the centre of each throat. Although these holes are empty, the accompanying drawings provide hopeful visions of what such damaged bodies can produce: one image portrays a yellow flower emerging from an open throat while another shows a red balloon that floats above a fragmented throat as if filled with air. These works suggest that purposefully altered, hybrid bodies can produce unexpected, but not necessarily superior, opportunities for life.

Bachmann continues to explore the damaged throat in another work, reflecting on the loss of the ability to speak and laugh that can result from the treatment of head and neck cancer. Whereas people recovering from surgery must learn to talk in a different voice, this installation focuses on the listening performed by others. An oval, clay form rests on a small pedestal, conveying sounds that are at first unclear. Visitors are invited to lean over the sound piece, adjust their bodily comportment, and take the time to comprehend the sound of laughter. A related sculptural work similarly asks visitors to slow down and recognize difference, but offers silence rather than sound. Seven small, smooth stones have been carefully placed on a shelf, invoking a collector who imbues them with meaning. Viewers might notice that some of the stones are found objects, shaped by the repetitive motion of waves, while others have been molded by hand from clay. In keeping with other works by Bachmann, natural and cultural forms engage with each other, sometimes remaining at odds and sometimes becoming indistinguishable.

In *Familiar* (2016), Sean Caulfield creates another site of quiet contemplation, combining found photographs with medical imagery to consider the domestic spaces of illness and recovery. Nine large squares are arranged in three even rows to produce a grid pattern that extends above the viewers' eye level, drawing their attention to the architecture of the wall.

This spatial element is enhanced by the three narrow, wooden shelves on which the squares rest, leaning against the wall like decorative plates in a kitchen. The panels are composed of carefully selected visual fragments. Three squares include the same floral arrangement resting behind two tea cups to suggest a feminine realm of care and communication. Two other panels portray a decorated lamp hanging in a room with wallpaper that would now be considered outdated. Drained of colour, the black-, white-, and sepia-toned images seem to be from the past, recovered by someone striving to remember a history even as it fades away. The repetition of images reinforces this notion of returning to familiar spaces, though something else has been introduced. Those with medical knowledge might recognize the images of magnified cancer cells, while others could see them as a decorative element, like wallpaper or a patterned kitchen counter. A sheet of plexiglass protects each square and renders it more substantial, alluding to scientific specimens arranged on slides, but also signifying everyday utility. This combination of science and the mundane reveals the domestic realm as a key site of both medical care and tangible memory. The still life is central to this message because it has traditionally been linked with vibrant life, given as a gift to revive patients, but also associated with the ephemeral nature of all living things, reproduced as a sign of human mortality. Even as viewers are invited to rest with this commonplace image, any sense of ease cannot last long for there is no straightforward connection between the panels, no way to make them coalesce into a single message.

Bradley Necyk's installation, *Waiting Room* (2016), uses video technologies to make time palpable, creating a sense of anticipation. Two large TV screens project fragmented human faces. The pieces separate and rejoin without ever forming a coherent person or conventional portrait. This lack of resolution is unsettling, especially since the sections are in constant motion, portraying the face as a grotesque mask that floats and remains unmoored. To make this work, the artist videotaped collaborators, including people recovering from head and neck cancer, as they sat in front of a green screen, moving their head and upper body at will. Manipulating a rotobrush editing tool, Necyk cut out sections of each face—forehead, nose, iris, jaw, lips—frame by frame, offsetting thousands of them in layers that move independently of each other. This intensive, time-consuming method recalls the surgical approach employed by Ho-You, while referencing the digital technologies used by medical experts to assess patients, collecting the information needed to disassemble and then restore their faces. *Waiting Room* recognizes the disorienting experiences of head and neck cancer patients as they are transformed. Those who view the video installation and

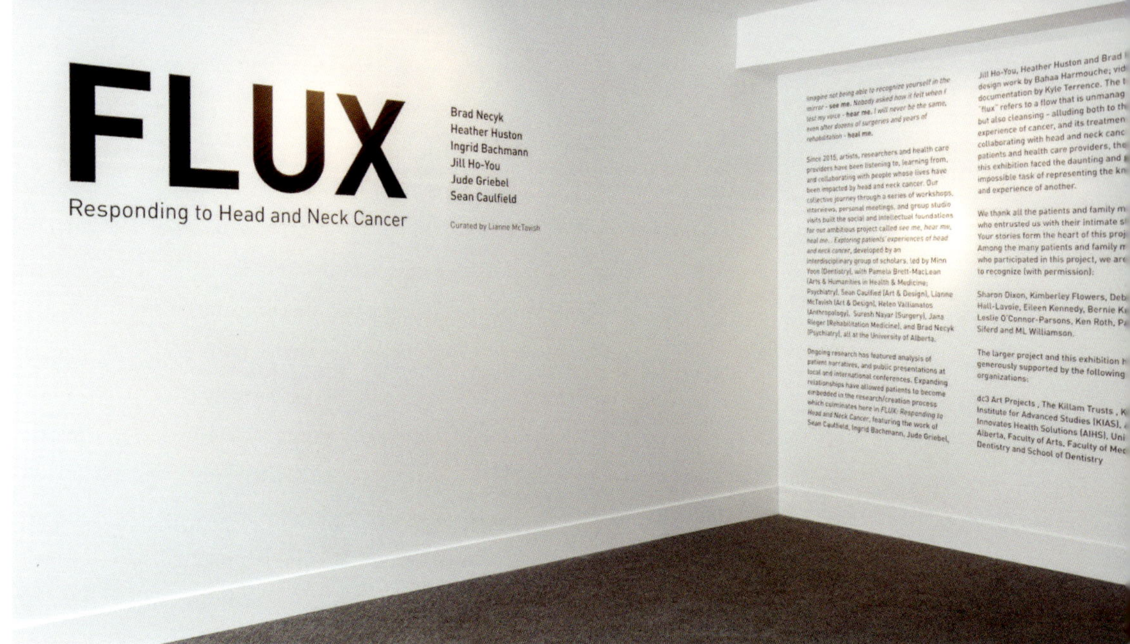

FLUX: Responding to Head and Neck Cancer *exhibition introductory signage at dc3 Art Projects, Edmonton, AB.* Photo: Blaine Campbell

its accompanying light boxes are invited to sympathize with these patients, responding in visceral ways to the continual and potentially nauseating movement on the screens. At the same time, these viewers are separated from the activity on the screens, positioned as perpetual outsiders. In the end, those who have not undergone invasive medical procedures can never fully comprehend and feel the fragmentation of identity that impacts people recovering from head and neck cancer.

The title of Heather Huston's installation, *I Am Wearing Clothes, but I Am Naked* (2016), directly quotes a collaborator recovering from laryngeal cancer, describing his vulnerability while in public situations. Huston strives to represent the ways in which disease alters everyday encounters, limiting social interaction. Rather than focusing on such dramatic events as the announcement of a diagnosis or the experience of surgical procedures, her work considers their aftermath, when cancer has been "beaten" and regular life supposedly resumes. Layered photographs of two people, one male and one female, hang side by side on a wall. The life-sized figures remain apart, appearing to sit at the separate tables placed in front of them. A restaurant-grade plate rests on each table. The plates are empty, but strangely decorated with hands at once beautiful and grotesquely overtaken by foliage. These hands gesture hesitantly, as if reaching for connection. The wooden tables sprout tree branches and other organic forms to magnify the sense that something is not quite right. Dis-ease is also reinforced in the portraits, which are difficult to read because they are covered in hand-drawn lines and arrows that suggest medical measurement and decision-making. The human figures are practically invisible beneath these layers of mark-making, potentially reduced to sites of information rather than individuality. By placing these altered figures in a lonely social setting, the artist responded to recovering head and neck cancer patient descriptions of the difficulties of eating and drinking post-treatment. Activities previously linked with pleasure and the development of relationships became burdensome necessities often done alone. Though not featured in fundraising campaigns or inspiring stories of survival, the permanent transformation of social encounters is part of the lived reality of those recovering from head and neck cancer.

The works featured in the FLUX exhibition are united in their dedication to exploring, representing, and recreating the stories, experiences, and embodied knowledge of people recovering from head and neck cancer. All six artists have thoughtfully and imaginatively provided new ways to think about and understand head and neck cancer, without attempting to simplify or sanitize this disease and its impact. The range of responses, materials, and formats on display indicates the complexity of this topic and the multiple reactions it can provoke. In addition to respecting the varied paths of people undergoing cancer treatment, FLUX acknowledges that different visitors will bring their own bodies and histories to the exhibition, providing them with open-ended questions rather than easily digested answers. In keeping with the overall theme of flux, this collaborative, interdisciplinary, and interactive exhibition shows that human bodies are enduring and malleable, subject to disaster but also to repair.

Bradley Necyk

For me, this project was about trust. Over the course of many months and numerous meetings with patients involved in the project, I learned that head and neck cancer is neither something that you get past, nor a battle you win. For those in recovery, *survivor* is an inadequate label. These individuals fight a never-ending battle, from the traumatic event of diagnosis and rupture of one's sense of self and identity, through to the tests, scans, waiting rooms, radiation, chemotherapy, surgeries, reconstruction, physiotherapy, prosthetics, more waiting rooms, and, for some, return of cancer. You find yourself in a continual state of "doing-illness."

I began to appreciate that there is an art to doing-illness that involves constant engagement with the health system, bodily discipline, support networks, and, for some, a new relationship between themselves and illness—an integration, an acceptance. However, one's way

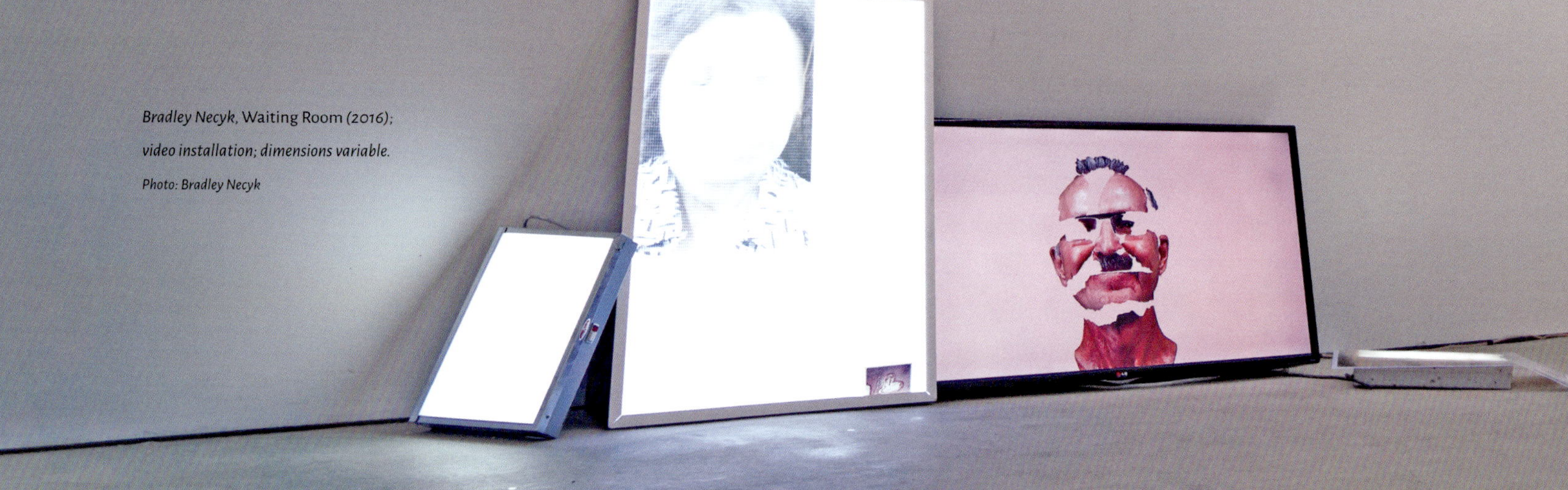

Bradley Necyk, Waiting Room *(2016); video installation; dimensions variable. Photo: Bradley Necyk*

of being in the world is dramatically unmoored. Many examples of this disruptive unmooring were shared with me. They ranged from the obvious and painful—losing the ability to work, and watching social relationships shift and change in response to the illness—to the intimately personal—experiencing changes in the way the body moves, speaks, and eats.

The trust that developed among all the participants in this project allowed me to gain a deeper understanding of what doing-illness means—of the trauma that begins with diagnosis and continues through treatment, but does not end there. Post-treatment, the trauma persists as a dizzying dislocation of the self in relation to its own corporeal body. This is the tough narrative, rooted in trust, that I was able to explore with my artwork.

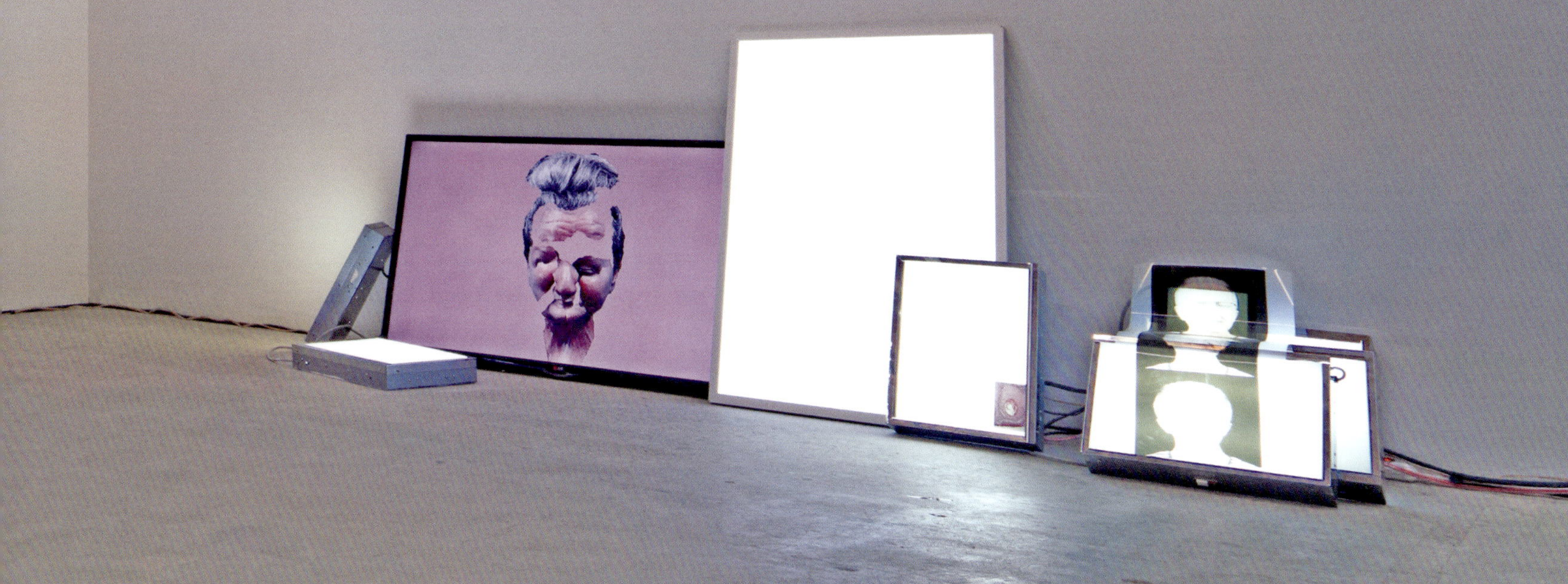

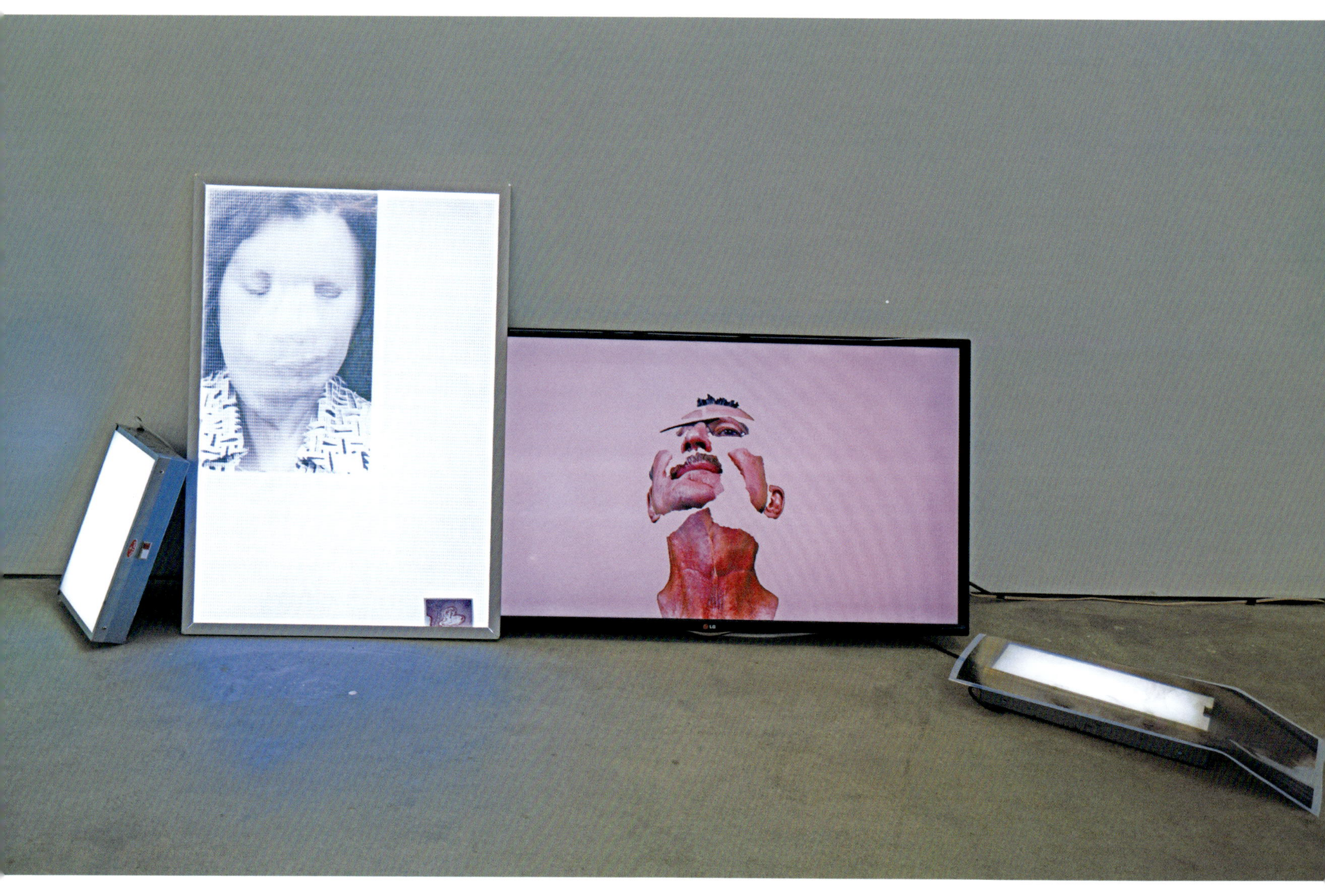

Bradley Necyk, details of Waiting Room *(2016). Photo: Bradley Necyk*

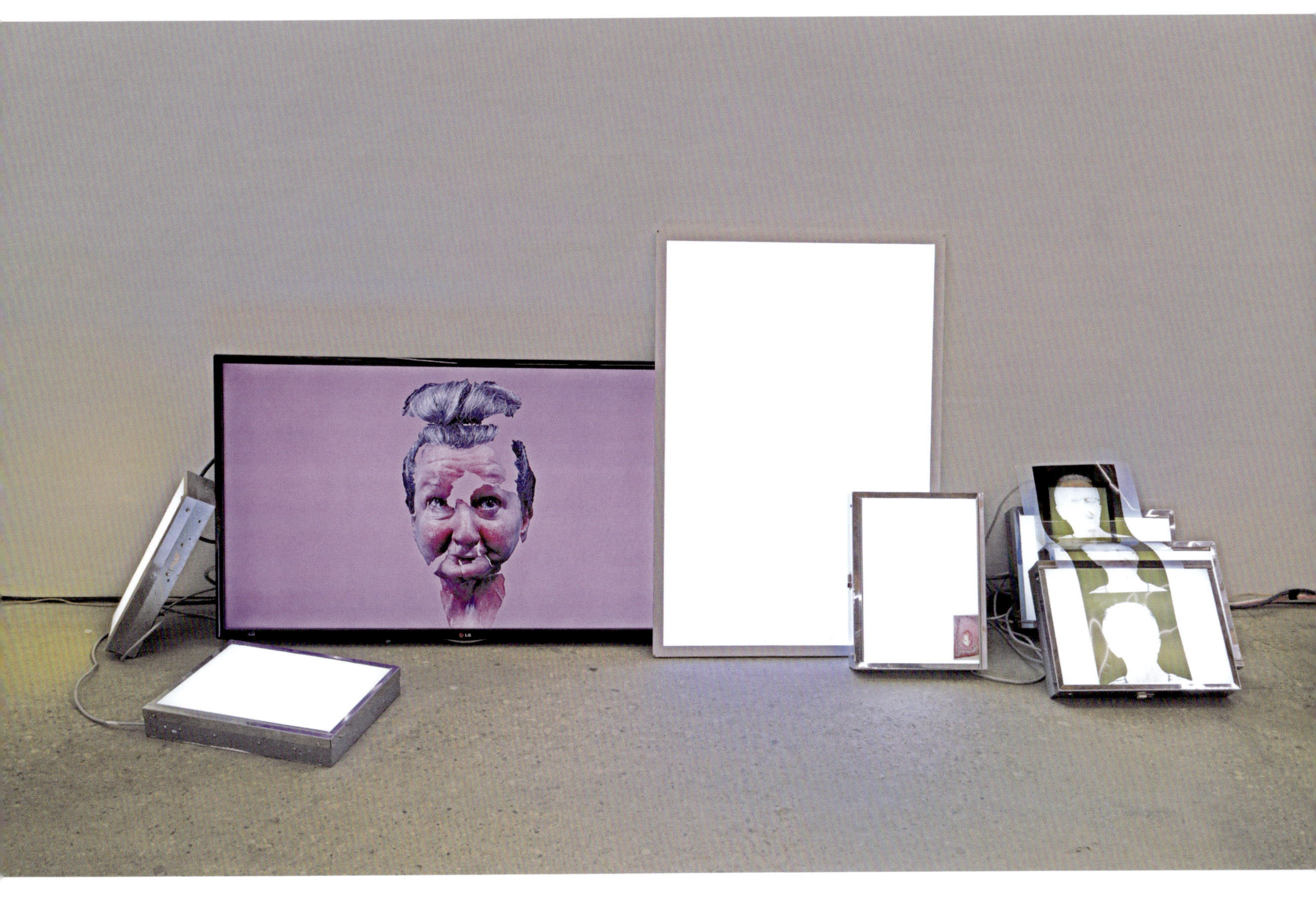

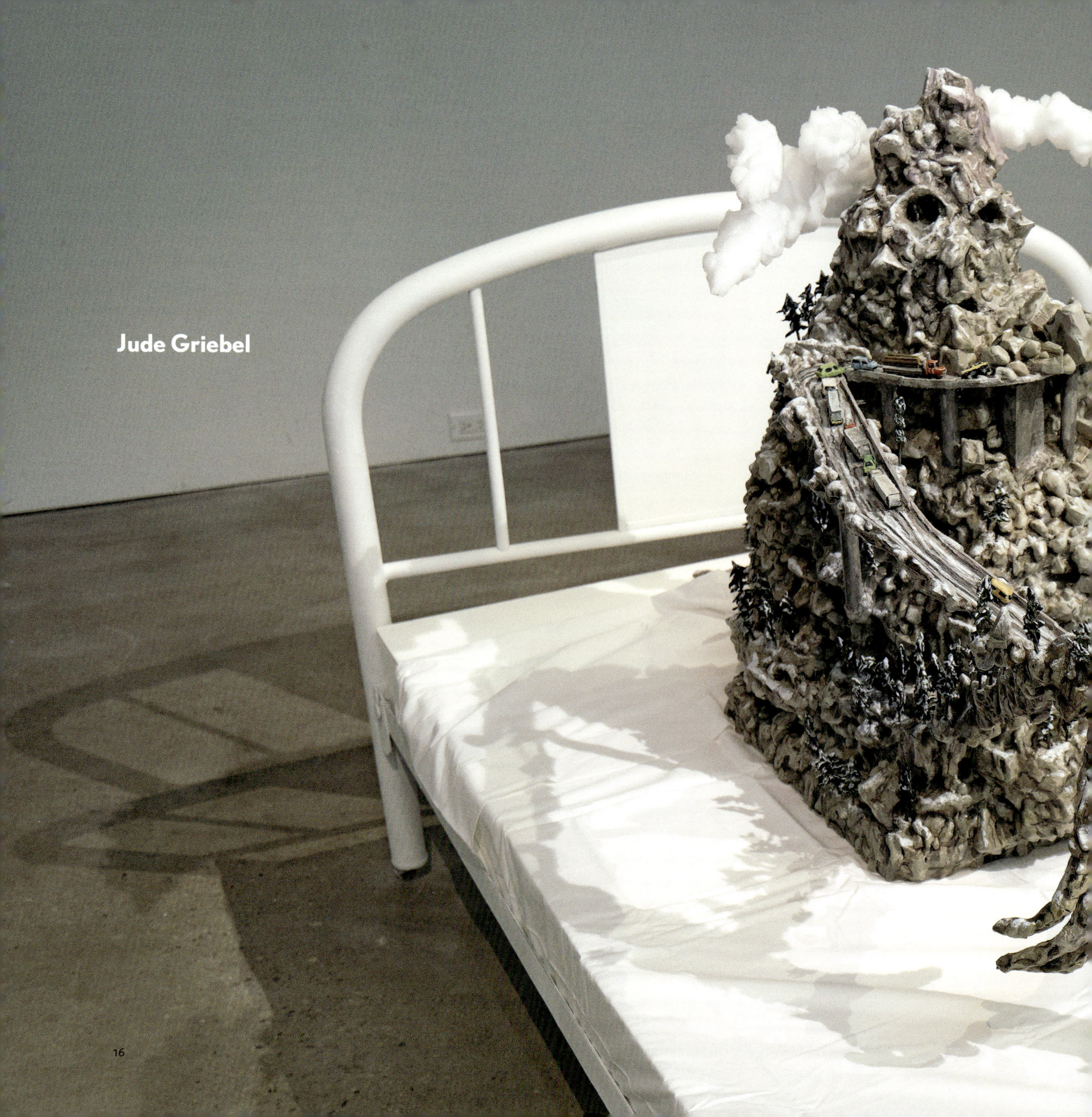

Jude Griebel

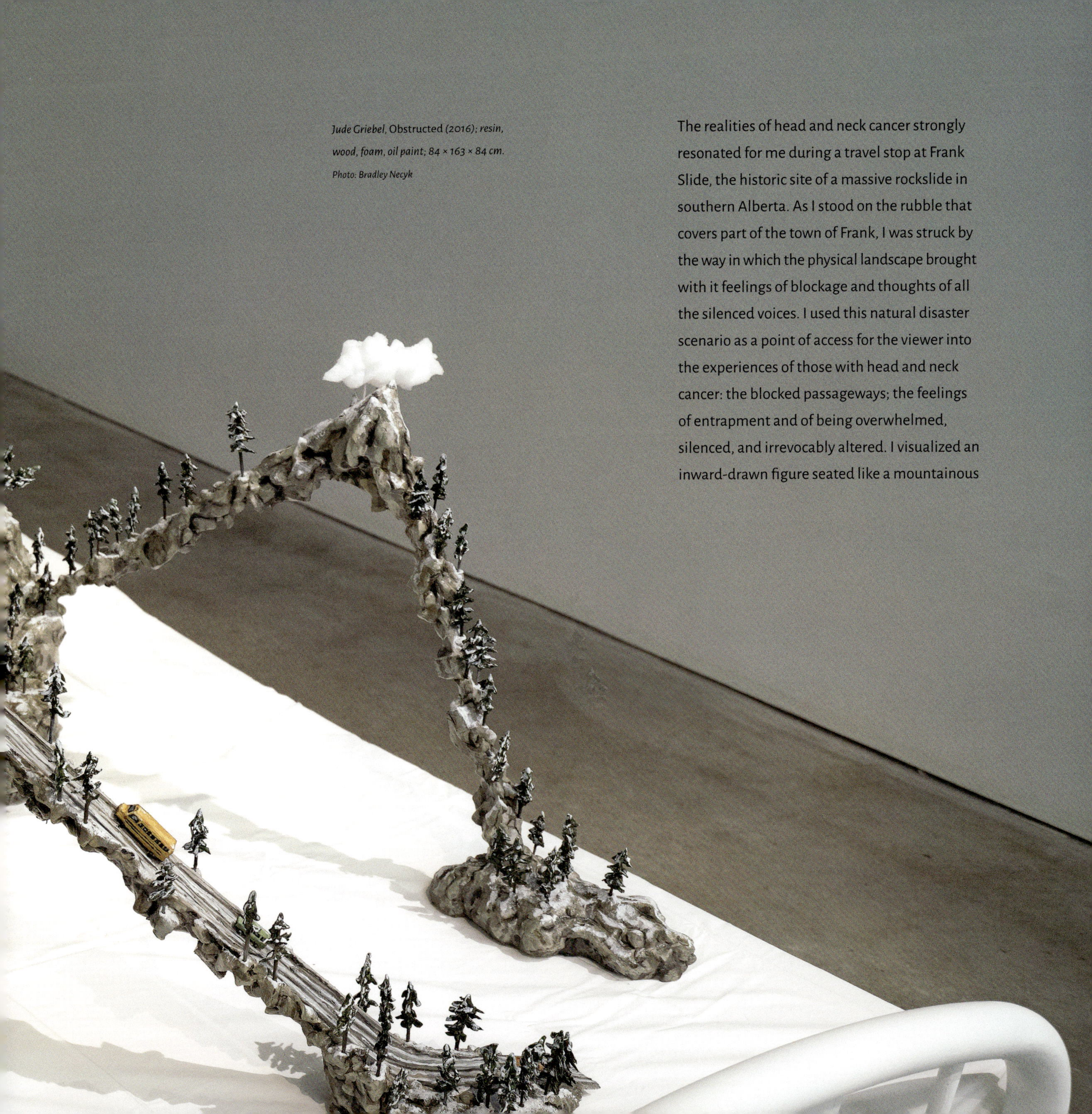

Jude Griebel, Obstructed (2016); resin, wood, foam, oil paint; 84 × 163 × 84 cm. Photo: Bradley Necyk

The realities of head and neck cancer strongly resonated for me during a travel stop at Frank Slide, the historic site of a massive rockslide in southern Alberta. As I stood on the rubble that covers part of the town of Frank, I was struck by the way in which the physical landscape brought with it feelings of blockage and thoughts of all the silenced voices. I used this natural disaster scenario as a point of access for the viewer into the experiences of those with head and neck cancer: the blocked passageways; the feelings of entrapment and of being overwhelmed, silenced, and irrevocably altered. I visualized an inward-drawn figure seated like a mountainous

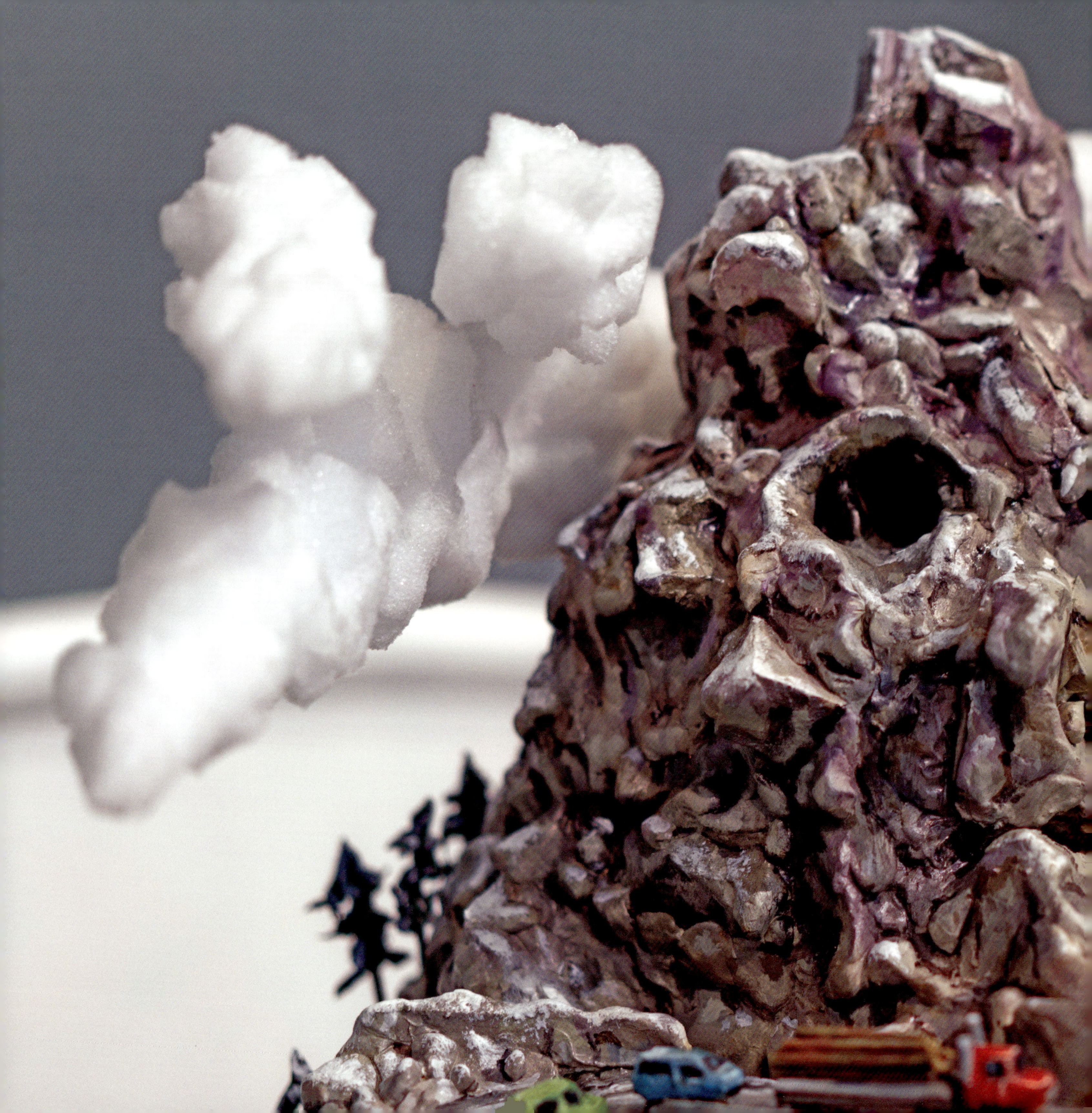

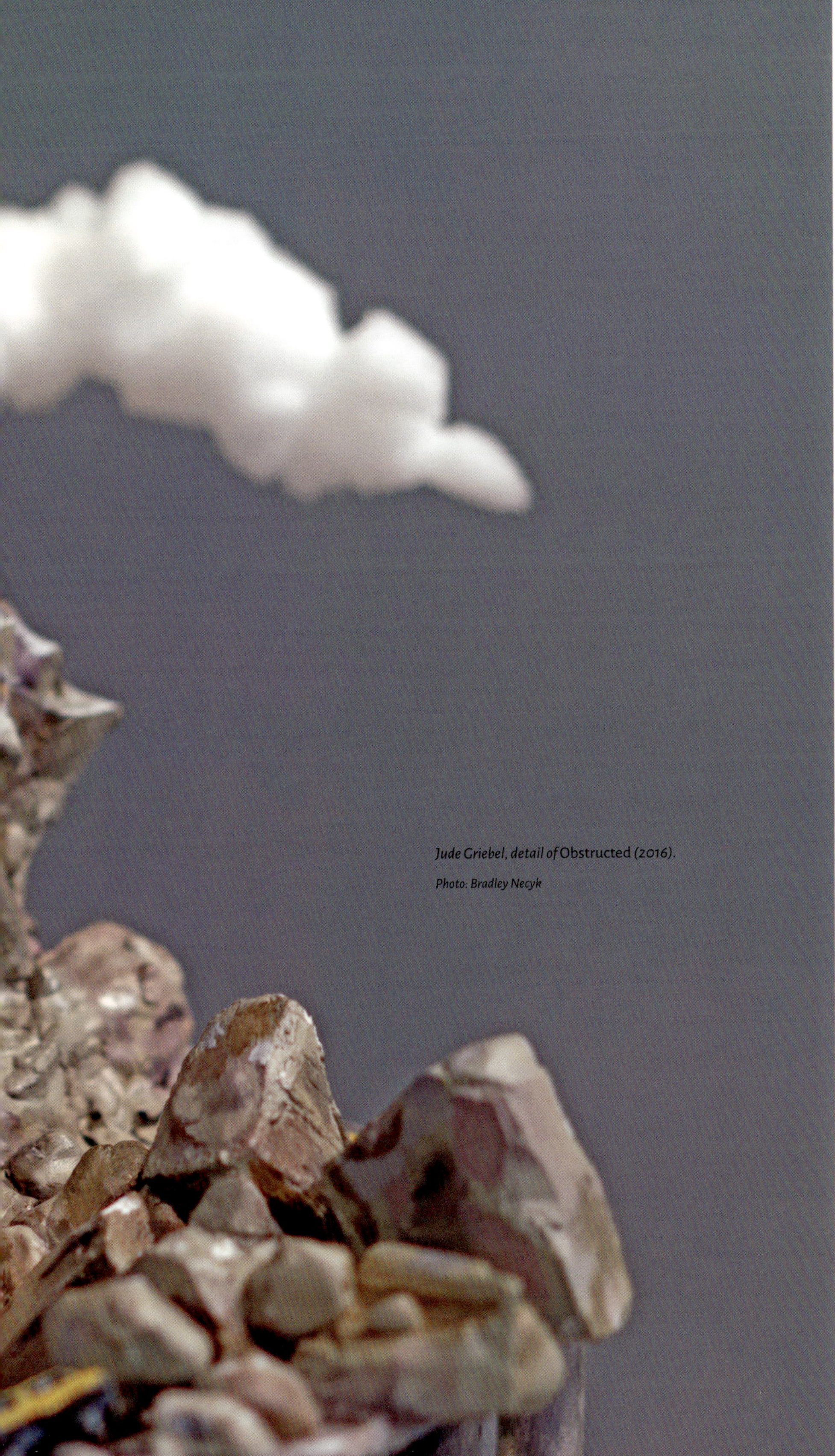

Jude Griebel, detail of Obstructed *(2016).*

Photo: Bradley Necyk

landscape, with a bowed head as its highest elevation. A landslide over a road traversing its throat became a dramatic, symbolic way of addressing the urgent and unexpected arrival of head and neck cancer. The mountainous figure's throat is a two-lane highway where nourishment, air, and words once traveled.

We seldom hear, in medical and disaster narratives, individual accounts of struggle from those who were there, who lived the experience: The buried miners who burrowed their way to the surface through coal seams. The patients who emerge from the darkened tunnels of their head and neck cancer journey scarred, reassembled, often lacking voices—alive, yet transformed. As these narratives are buried in traditional accounts of medicine and culture, perhaps there are metaphorical ways in which disasters might be used to highlight individual patient experience. My sculptural work attempts to form connections between personal urgency and the universal impact of a shifting environment.

Suresh Nayar & Bernie Krewski

A (High Wire) Dance

Editors' Introduction

Suresh Nayar (roman text) and Bernie Krewski (italic text) wrote this essay together to demonstrate their parallel yet distinctive experiences of head and neck cancer. Krewski, a cancer patient diagnosed 15 years ago, met Nayar, a prosthodontist, when he was referred for treatment at the Institute for Reconstructive Sciences in Medicine (iRSM; Edmonton, AB), in a clinical context. In this essay, the authors reflect on how they developed a collaborative relationship, learning from each other while negotiating the uncertainties that adhere to the treatment of and recovery from a serious illness.

Clinician

There is a general perception that clinicians at the coalface of cancer patient treatment and care are used to dealing with the vagaries of the disease and its effects, including the mortality associated with it. That perception is valid and compelling, but it reflects only one aspect of our working lives.

Working with cancer patients is rewarding. It is also complex, challenging, and marked by frequent uncertainties. Often, it is like dancing on a high wire, an image evoked in Miriam Mandel's poem "Encore": "I dance a high wire / with no net to catch me."[1]

A clinician is expected to sense what a patient is going through and to empathize. That, however, has to be reconciled with a basic, professional principle of medical care: to sufficiently distance oneself from the situation in order to discharge one's duties as objectively as possible. Thus, as a prosthodontist, I dance on a high wire daily.

Patient

It is common for people to think that patients referred to centres like the iRSM can look forward, after treatment, to returning to their previous way of life. The current marvels of bodily reconstruction offer hope and can bring about much needed comfort and relief. However, reconstructive outcomes are often precarious and unpredictable.

When I was referred to the iRSM, much had already occurred that had demonstrably changed my life. I, too, was dancing on a very high wire. I recall wondering, What if reconstructive surgery does not improve my quality of life?

What do clinicians expect of patients? The current trend is to involve patients in making decisions about what treatments to consider. What do patients expect of themselves? Research suggests that many, if not most, patients want clinicians to decide what is best for them. Besides feeling overwhelmed, they are likely to say they have insufficient medical knowledge to make decisions about treatment. That is the high wire on which patients often walk.

My professional responsibility is to reconstruct and restore. However, the variables of the disease and the effect of treatment are such that the prospects for many patients may be bleak. This is something that I have to deal with constantly.

The diagnosis of cancer can be mind-numbing to patients. At the moment of diagnosis, they find themselves at a crossroads with many paths to choose from, including declining further treatment. Fear of the unknown is upon them and making a decision becomes demanding. At times they want me to decide for them, which I cannot—but their struggle puts me in a dilemma: As a clinician, I must keep a sufficient distance. But I am a human. I have emotions. How much of my own experience can I, and should I, reveal?

Although this dance is inevitably precarious, I love the artistic and creative aspect of my work, and what I am able to accomplish. As for the patients, I know that sometimes even the smallest amount of surgical reconstruction amounts to a very large improvement. I can see in their eyes, faces, and smiles—some of which have gone through this restorative work—how much it, and the restored function it offers, means to them. And it is, moreover, meaningful to their family members—and to me!

Treating head and neck cancer generally involves a greater number of health disciplines than any other type of cancer. Not surprisingly, my accomplishments as a prosthodontist are

If, as a patient, I leave decisions about treatment in the hands of the clinicians, what happens if the results do not turn out as anticipated? Am I further burdened with being responsible for these results? Should I show or even express my disappointment, realizing that I did have a choice but was too frightened to make it?

When someone is diagnosed with cancer, the word that, even if it is not said out loud, rings most clearly in their ears—and those of their family and friends—is death. *The stress and anxiety of receiving a cancer diagnosis impacts one's ability to absorb and make sense of information shared by clinicians. My approach was to manage my fear of whether I was going to live, or whether my life would soon be coming to an end.*

At this point, I was incapable of deciding anything. I wanted the medical specialists to decide—they have the expertise. I wondered, Are they aware of my emotional turmoil? Should I tell them how frightened I am?

After seven difficult years recovering from radiation treatments, two major surgeries, loss of speech for a year, extracted teeth, and living with a disfigured face, I arrived at the IRSM in early 2014 to be assessed for dental implants. The problem soon became obvious: It was not at all clear that implants could even be inserted into my radiated jaws that only half opened.

In an early appointment during the complicated assessment process, I asked Dr. Suresh Nayar whether there were any artists in his family. Looking puzzled, he replied there were none. By then I had noticed, amidst measurements and many oral photographs, the artistry involved in dental restoration.

based on teamwork. I am simply a member of a team and their contributions are often equal to, or more than, mine.

Sometimes I envy artists. What they do is usually displayed and exhibited. It is publicly admired. If people happen to not like a piece of art, they can walk away. Insofar as my work is a similarly creative process, I would like to be like them. But my work also involves treating a person with feelings and emotions. That makes things challenging when treatment outcomes differ from what a patient had imagined or expected.

Dealing with the challenges and risks involved in reconstructive work is profoundly worthwhile, particularly when it transforms a patient's life. Having said all of this, I will continue to dance on a high wire!

NOTE

1. Mandel, M. (1974). Encore. *Branching Out*, 1(1), 42.

Dr. Nayar, besides applying medical science, was also an artist.

What I find so admirable about artists is their ability to create an object or a piece of music that is unique to them, and seldom exactly copied. Equally, if not more commendable, is the skillful and adroit work of clinicians, acknowledging the distinctiveness and individuality of each patient.

Like artists, clinicians often work in relative silence. They know what steps typically need to be taken, and might be achieved by the end of the treatments. But the condition of every patient's body is different, and the process can be marked by uncertainties. There is no guarantee that the result will be as planned.

Such risk factors, fortunately, were not conveyed to me as I experienced multiple impressions of my mouth. The first oral surgery involved bone grafting followed by 20 hours in an oxygen chamber to prevent infection, then by several months of healing. Next, there were more impressions to prepare for a second surgery to install the foundational hardware for the implants—and more time for healing.

What was striking, as I sat in a dental chair for dozens of hours, was that healing was occurring far beyond its physical aspects. The compassionate care I received from Dr. Nayar and his colleagues for so many months was so consistent and remarkable. They made my life seem so indelibly normal. Past times of suffering were slowly being forgotten.

The eventual result of the surgeries—a set of teeth that fit me—created a renewed sense of self. I now dance on a high wire with a new sense of identity.

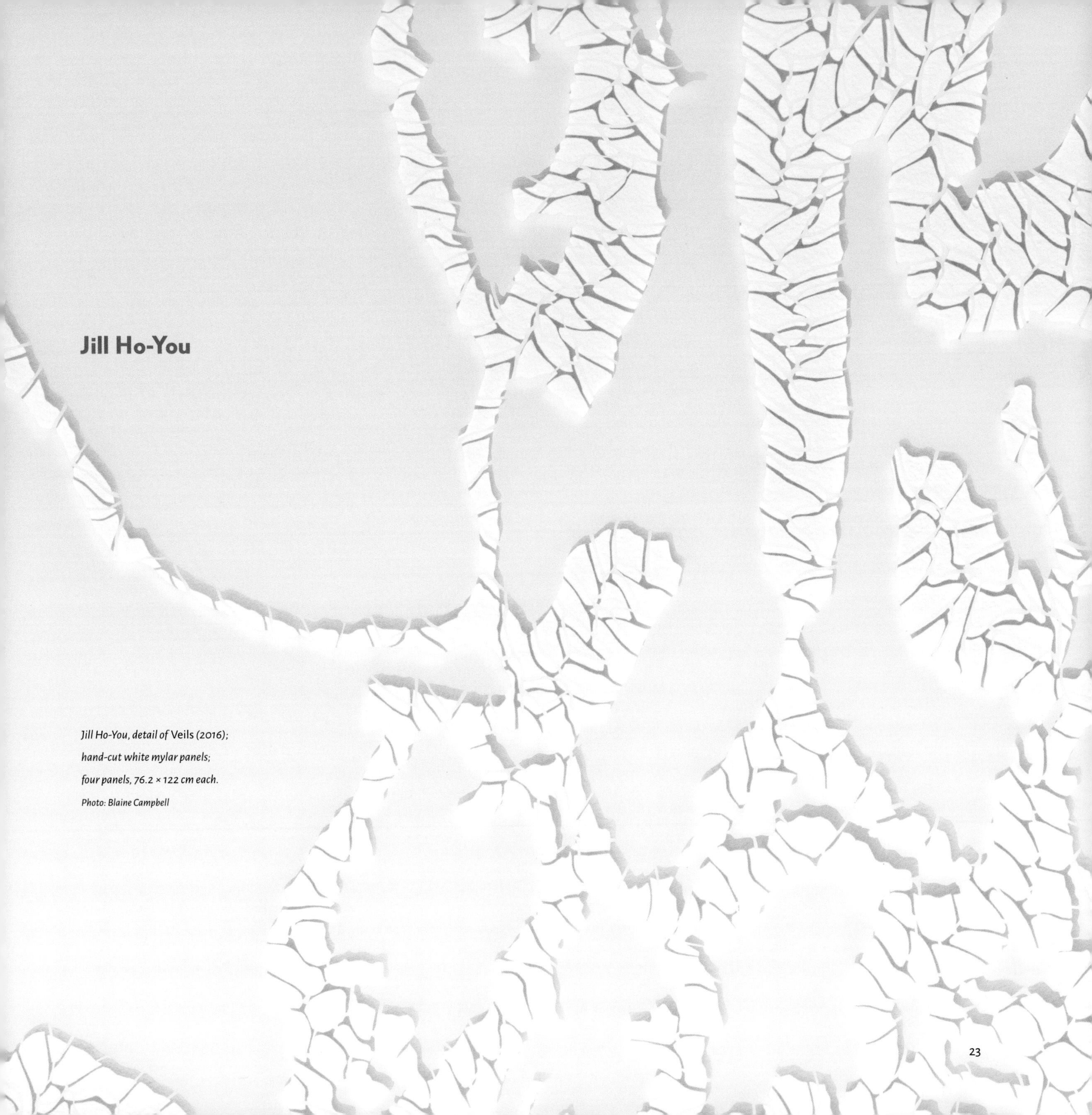

Jill Ho-You

Jill Ho-You, detail of Veils *(2016); hand-cut white mylar panels; four panels, 76.2 × 122 cm each.*

Photo: Blaine Campbell

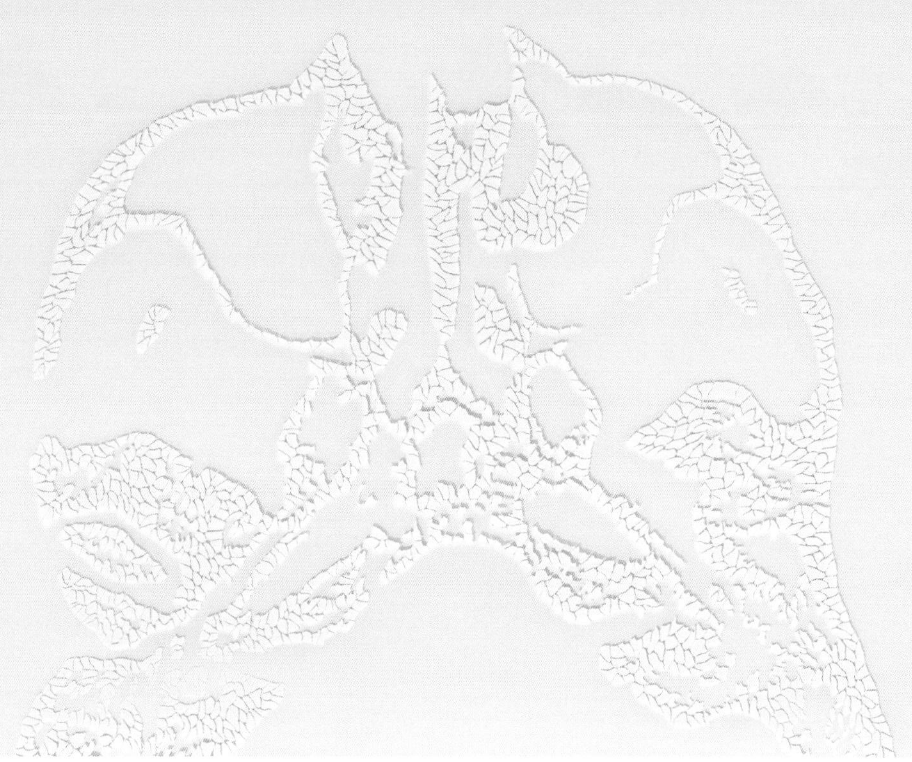

As an artist, much of my work has focused on exploring connections between identity, memory, and the body. Over the course of this project, the conversations I have had with people who have been treated for head and neck cancer, along with their family members and the medical clinicians involved in their care, have reinforced and heightened my awareness of the fine line that exists between health and illness. Our conversations have also deepened my awareness of the multiple, complex, unimagined decisions that must be negotiated over the course of treatment and rehabilitation. The fact that the body can endure serious illness along with extended, grueling medical treatments including painful reconstructions that take years to complete speaks both to the resiliency of the human body and to advancements in medical science. Learning the details of treatment and hearing our collaborators speak to their subsequent struggles also highlighted their psychological and emotional strength and endurance.

I wanted my piece to highlight both the physical and psychological fragility and strength of those affected by head and neck cancer, and also recognize the enormous role of time in the process of treatment and recovery. By transforming patient CT scans into intricate, labour-intensive physical objects, I allude to the long, uncertain path on which head and neck cancer patients and their families must embark.

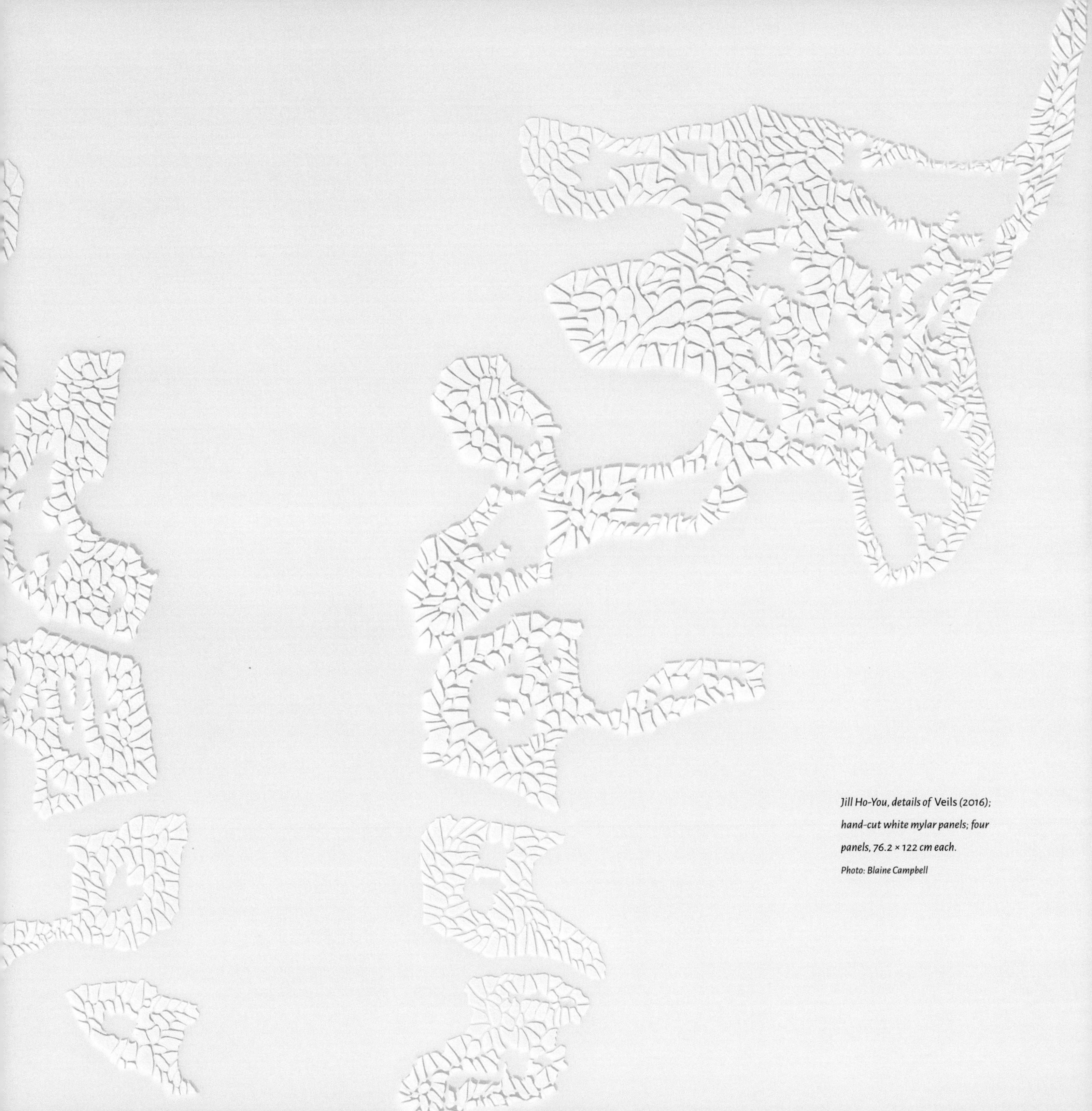

Jill Ho-You, details of Veils *(2016); hand-cut white mylar panels; four panels, 76.2 × 122 cm each.*

Photo: Blaine Campbell

Heather Huston

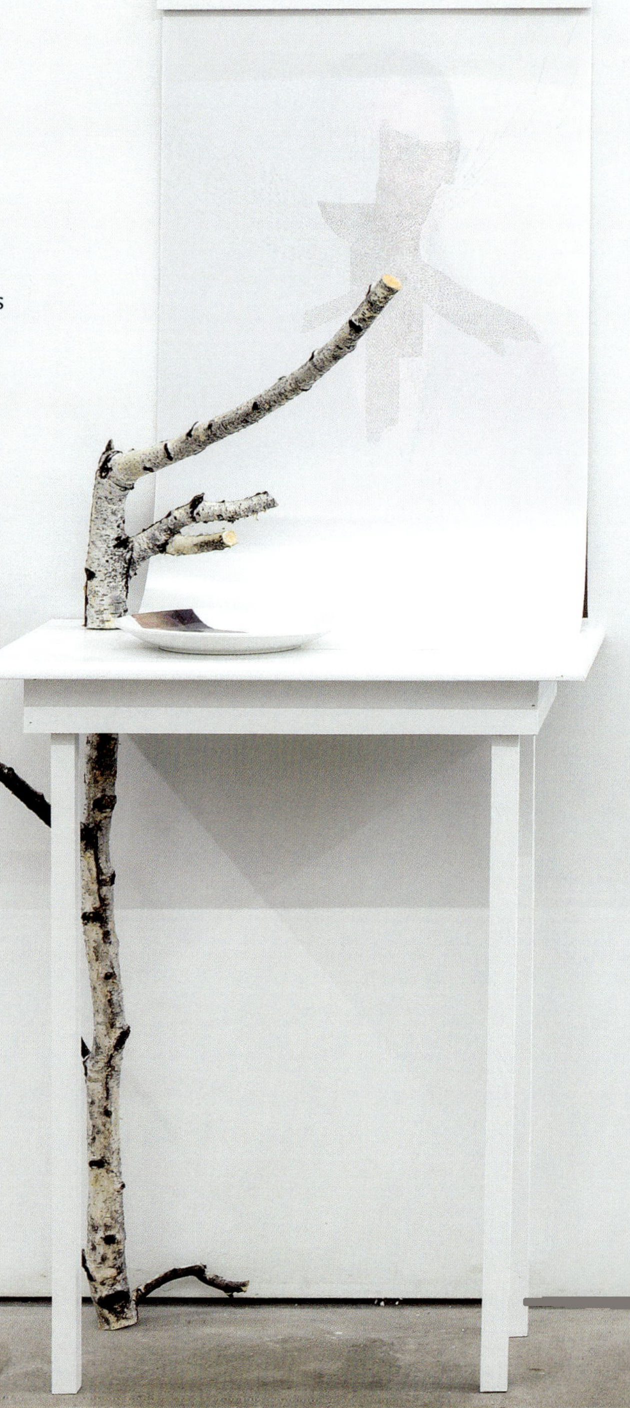

Over the past few years, my artistic research has focused on exploring how we understand the body through both medical data and personal experience. I have used my own subjective experiences as a starting point for these inquiries. This project afforded me the opportunity to expand on my research through the lens of other people's stories and narratives. It was both challenging and inspiring to translate the complex process associated with a diagnosis of head and neck cancer, the many subsequent treatments, and the ongoing recovery.

I experienced the patients and family members who participated in this project as acutely self-aware, passionate, and highly articulate. In addition to the physical devastation of head and neck cancer, they openly shared the social and psychological impact of the disease during our many discussions and interviews. I was struck by the difficult and complex decisions regarding disfiguring and

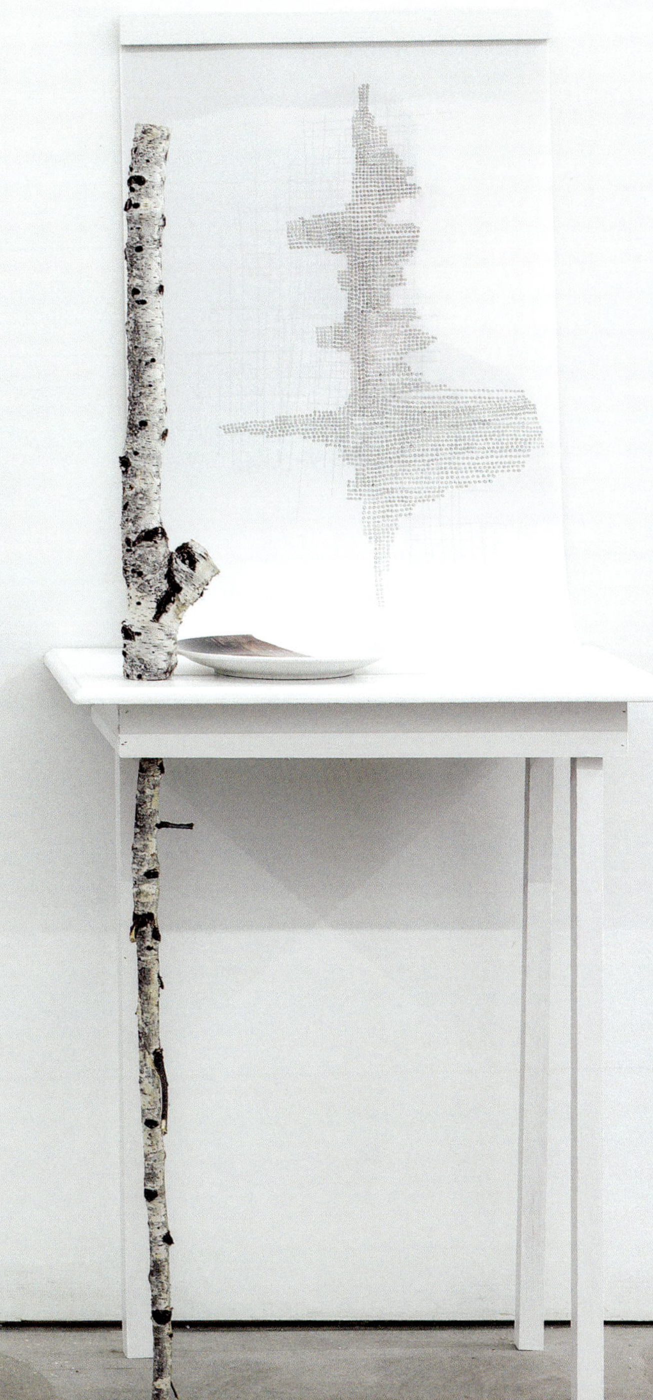

profoundly life-altering surgical procedures that patients face soon after receiving their diagnosis. I was especially affected by the impact of head and neck cancer treatment on social dimensions of eating: What for most is experienced as a pleasurable activity that connects people can, for head and neck cancer patients, become fraught, distressing, and sometimes impossible.

I wanted my work to reflect the complex challenges faced by people who have been affected by head and neck cancer as they navigate the distance created by their previous, familiar lives, and their current ones.

Heather Huston, I Am Wearing Clothes, but I Am Naked *(2016); digital print on paper, pencil on vellum, decals on ceramic plates, wooden tree branches;* 183 × 152 × 38 cm.
Photo: Blaine Campbell

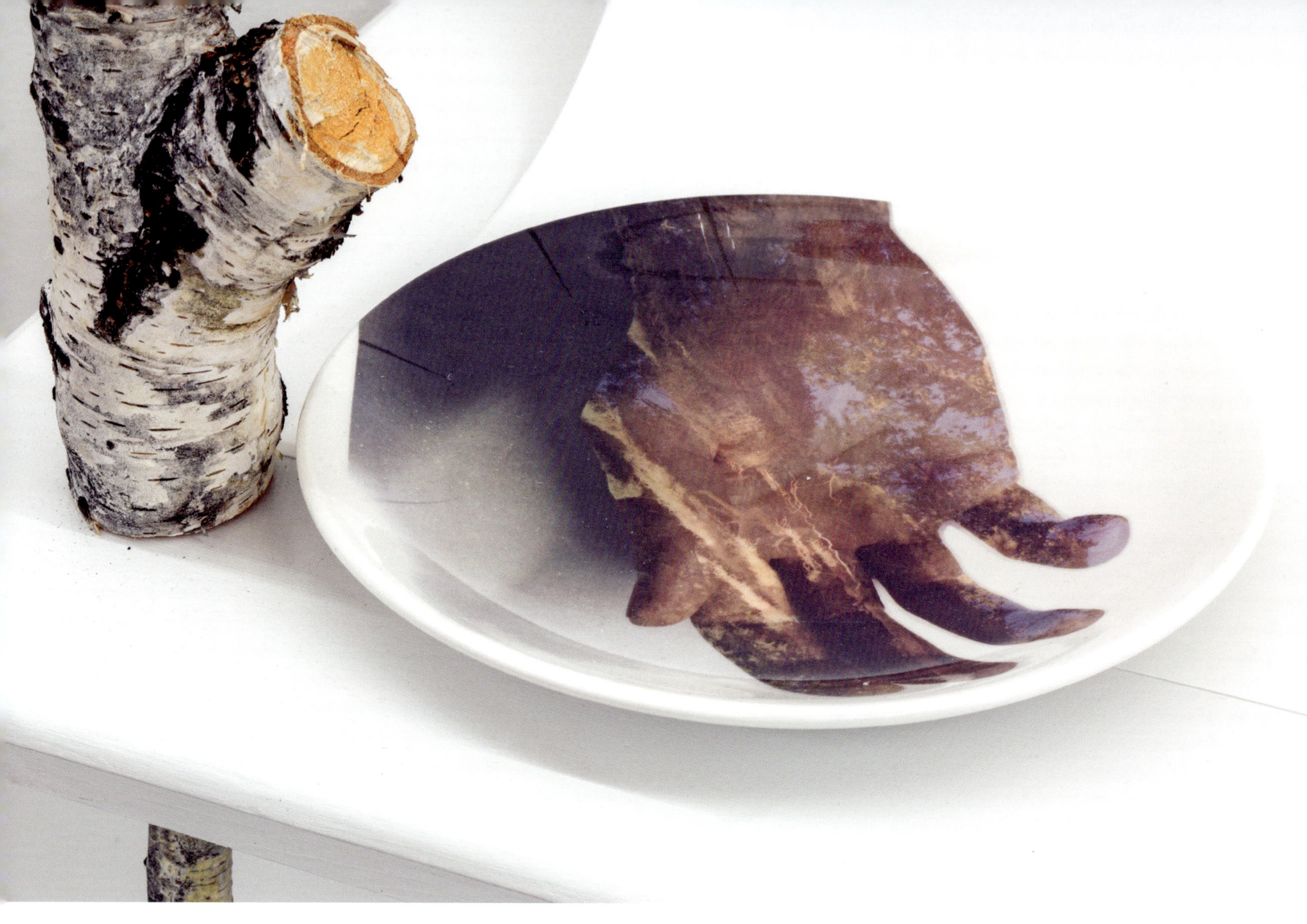

Heather Huston, detail of I Am Wearing Clothes, but I Am Naked *(2016). Photo: Blaine Campbell*

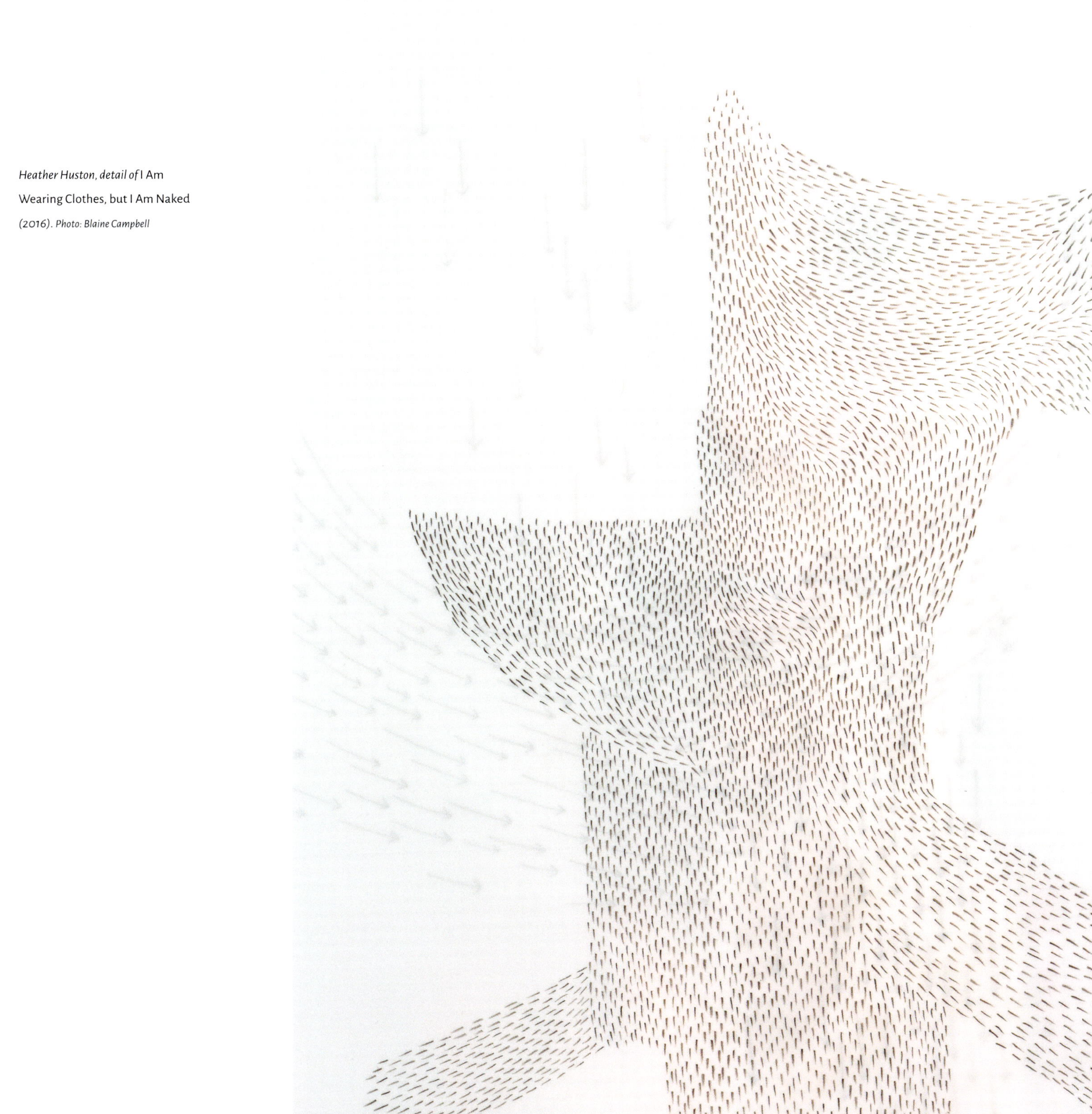

Heather Huston, detail of I Am Wearing Clothes, but I Am Naked *(2016). Photo: Blaine Campbell*

Helen Vallianatos

Feeding New Selves

Dis-moi ce que tu manges, je te dirai ce que tu es.
[Tell me what you eat and I will tell you what you are.]

—A. BRILLAT-SAVARIN (1825), *Physiologie du goût, ou méditations de gastronomie transcendante.*

Food serves to mark our identities. Through eating, we imbibe objects that are full of social meanings and that reveal our place in the world. For instance, in many cultures, certain foods are associated with men, other foods with women. In North America, light foods such as salads tend to be associated with women while heavy, hearty food (for example, "Hungry Man" frozen dinners) are associated more with men.[1] Food can also be used to indicate social status ("high" cuisine versus "poor people's foods"), and social group affiliation (halal or kosher foods, for example).[2] Learning what to eat and formulating sensory and aesthetic taste preferences happens continually from birth as part of the process of socialization. Consequently, food and taste practices become "natural," part of our everyday routines that we take for granted. At the same time, they reflect our values and beliefs.[3] But what happens when one can no longer consume the foods that had marked their identity? Such is the case for most head and neck cancer survivors, many of whom must relearn how to swallow, let alone eat.

Many of the individuals who participated in the "see me, hear me, heal me" project required various degrees of tongue reconstruction in addition to alterations that affected the upper palate, jaw, and teeth. For many, their ability to chew and swallow food was significantly impaired. One participant noted, for example: "I would be trying to put this food down, and it would keep getting lodged in my throat...It would be coming out my nose and my mouth, and it was just horrible. I was having troubles even drinking Ensure."

Another participant, who also shared the challenges of eating post-surgery, echoed this:

> *Slowly, slowly we tried to—I had to do exercises, swallowing exercises. I was unable to swallow. A baby spoon of water wouldn't go down. And then they tried—I had to do all these swallowing exercises and then they tried to get me on Jell-O because I was unable to get [anything else] down without it going down the wrong way. And then slowly, slowly I was able to get just the tip of a teaspoon full of Jell-O. It had to be in one lump; then I was able to get it down. It slipped down. And that took weeks, and then it was pudding and then it was oats, porridge, and then slowly, slowly we worked it up to pureed foods, and it took almost a half a year to get me back to swallowing pureed foods.*

For this patient, eating—an activity that is necessary for survival and that, pre-treatment, was generally enjoyable—was dramatically altered. Transformed into a fearful process, eating required diligence, care, and concentrated attention to effect a careful, rhythmic balance between swallowing and breathing, and to safeguard against choking.

For others, relearning to swallow, and in turn eat, was less problematic, as their surgeries did not require removal of large portions of their tongue. One participant who had relatively little reconstruction, noted:

> *I just chew it, like an excessive amount more than usual because otherwise it just won't go down and it'll just come back up, and some of the—like the prescription medication that I take, it has to be like elongated. It can't be round because I can't actually take that down. It'll just come back up. It'll get stuck. And after I eat and drink I have to stay in the upright position, otherwise it just kind of comes up because there's nothing that will stop it from coming up.*

Even when patients experience less invasive oral procedures, they still need to be mindful of their eating to ensure food is swallowed and ingested.

Increased effort given to the process of eating does not lead to increased reward. In addition to the expended energy and attendant anxiety experienced, the ability to taste food is often altered post-surgery. If treatment required removal of the tongue (or parts thereof), taste buds are no longer present. For those who experience minimal or partial tongue reconstruction, radiation of oral cavities can also affect the sense of taste. Shifts in one's sense of taste can be confusing and disconcerting because of the role food, and tasting food, has in marking identities. Taste can refer not only to the sensation of taste, but also to aesthetics, where gustatory tastes demarcate social status.[4]

We symbolically construct our identity by consuming food and through our preferred and aspirational tastes.[5] What we eat becomes a part of us. We literally absorb what we consume. It is the sensory properties of food that allow for its poignant and powerful symbolic meanings. Through our senses, eating fosters social connections that transcend time and place, as illustrated by the power of comfort foods, or an immigrant's adherence to "food from the old country"[6]: just one whiff or taste of such foods evokes positive emotions and memories.

For head and neck cancer survivors, alterations in the sense of taste symbolize different selves before and after their cancer diagnosis, and particularly after surgery. As one participant noted, "My taste is gone. I can't distinguish between sweet and sour and spicy. If it's too spicy then it burns, by the way...taste, I don't have anymore. The thing that I can taste the best is coffee and I have this perfect taste in my mouth." This participant had spent almost two years unable to swallow and, perhaps because the taste of coffee remained, coffee became symbolic of bodily changes: "Every morning when I have my cup of coffee I enjoy every drop and every day it reminds me of those two years that I was unable to swallow anything at all and I appreciate everything that I can put in my mouth, and it would go down."

For this patient, sensitivity experienced in the mouth post-treatment meant that food, whether it was pureed or more akin to "regular" textures, needed to be bland. Spices, including salt and pepper, triggered painful sensations in and around the mouth. Other patients shared that imagined recollection of the taste of different foods developed over time, which helped them compensate for their altered ability to taste: "At first food was pretty bland, but now, you know, I've kind of gotten used to the taste. So I think I create the taste in my mind a lot more than what I actually get from my taste buds." This can be viewed as a coping process, with sensory memories, altered bodies, and new selves (re)connecting with ways of being or experiencing the world, attempting to (re)construct a sense of continuity across pre-diagnosis, and post-treatment periods.

Food is intensely personal. It sustains us. It is also a fundamental means of connecting with others and knowing one's place in the community and society. Commensality—eating and drinking together—is fundamental to human sociality. The profound changes that patients experienced in relation to their bodies and sense of selves is most poignantly illustrated in how their experience of head and neck cancer affected their ability to share meals. As one participant described, she still went out to eat with her husband, but "probably not as often as he'd like, because he says he feels bad we can't go out to eat and I can't eat and he sits there eating." She continued:

> *People look at him, and he goes, "I don't like that." ...I said, "Well, that's their problem," you know? But it's hard on him, you know? A lot of my friends don't know what to do, you know, because it's easy to go for coffee or—and I can't eat...I said, "I can still go for coffee. I can sit there and you can have the coffee and I can talk to you." So that's what we do now. So I've really had to work hard to stay normal.*

Eating and relishing in the taste of our food is a basic, uncomplicated experience that most of us take for granted—but for many head and neck cancer survivors, this is not the case.

The process of (re)learning how to swallow and eat is an ongoing one. Those who have been diagnosed with head and neck cancer continue to negotiate their understanding of themselves and their social relationships as they construct new identities and engage different social locations following treatment. While integral to self-nourishment, health, and healing, feeding one's new self often remains an intensely personal, hidden dimension of head and neck cancer.

NOTES

1. Counihan, C. (1999). *The anthropology of food and body: Gender, meaning and power*. New York: Routledge.
2. See Douglas, M. (1966). *Purity and danger: An analysis of concepts of pollution and taboo.* New York: Praeger; Goody, J. (1982). *Cooking, cuisine and class.* Cambridge: Cambridge University Press; Johnston, J. & Baumann, S. (2015). *Foodies: Democracy and distinction in the gourmet foodscape* (2nd ed.). New York: Routledge.
3. See Barthes, R. (2013). Towards a psychosociology of contemporary food consumption. In C. Counihan & P. Van Esterik (Eds.), *Food and society* (3rd ed., pp. 23–30). New York: Routledge; Bourdieu, P. (1984). *Distinction: A social critique of the judgment of taste*. Cambridge: Harvard University Press.
4. Korsmeyer, C. (1999). *Making sense of taste: Food and philosophy.* Ithaca: Cornell University Press.
5. Bourdieu (1984).
6. See Abdullah, N. (2016). Comfort food, memory and "home": Senses in transnational contexts. In D. Kalekin-Fishman & K.E.Y. Los (Eds.), *Everyday life in Asia: Social perspectives on the senses* (pp. 157–76). London: Routledge; Sutton, D. (2010). Food and the senses. *Annual Review of Anthropology, 39*, 209–23. https://doi.org/10.1146/annurev.anthro.012809.104957; Vallianatos, H. & Raine, K. (2008). Consuming food and constructing identities among Arabic and South Asian immigrant women. *Food, Culture & Society, 11*(3), 355–73. https://doi.org/10.2752/175174408X347900.

Sean Caulfield

Just before entering my second year of university, my mother, Ruth Caulfield, was diagnosed with head and neck cancer. This project gave me an opportunity to reflect on my experiences as my mother struggled with this illness and the impact of the treatment she received—treatment that ultimately extended her life, but that also brought disruption and hardships that impacted every aspect of daily life. Collaborating with patients, family members, and health care professionals fostered a sense of connection that enabled me to explore my memories in relation to others' experiences. Even after all the years that have passed since my mother confronted this illness, several overlapping and related stories emerged that led me to consider how illness transforms the routines of everyday life.

My mother's cancer imposed a kind of veil over my interactions with the world, distancing me from the normal routines of daily life—a phenomenon that I can only imagine was multiplied a hundredfold for my mother. Surprisingly, after treatment was complete, it was the everyday routines that became a source of support, solace, and healing. Simple, everyday acts—sitting together, listening to music, walking together—created a space in which the weight of constantly thinking about illness was temporarily relieved.

In *Familiar*, I have attempted to explore the multiple relational connections that exist between everyday domestic spaces and illness.

Sean Caulfield, Familiar *(2016); silkscreen on wood and plexiglass, wooden shelves; 203 × 203 cm. Photo: Blaine Campbell*

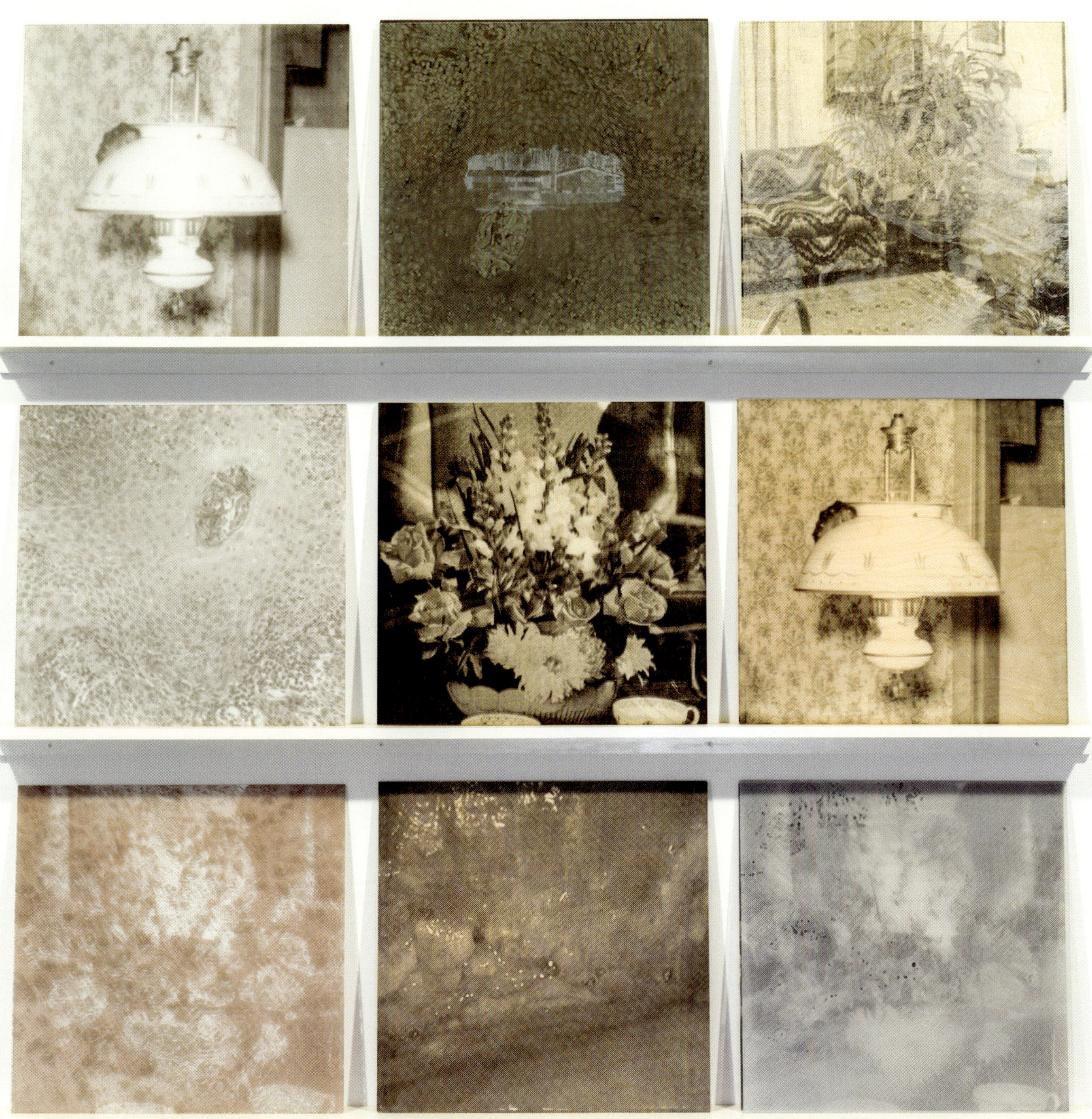

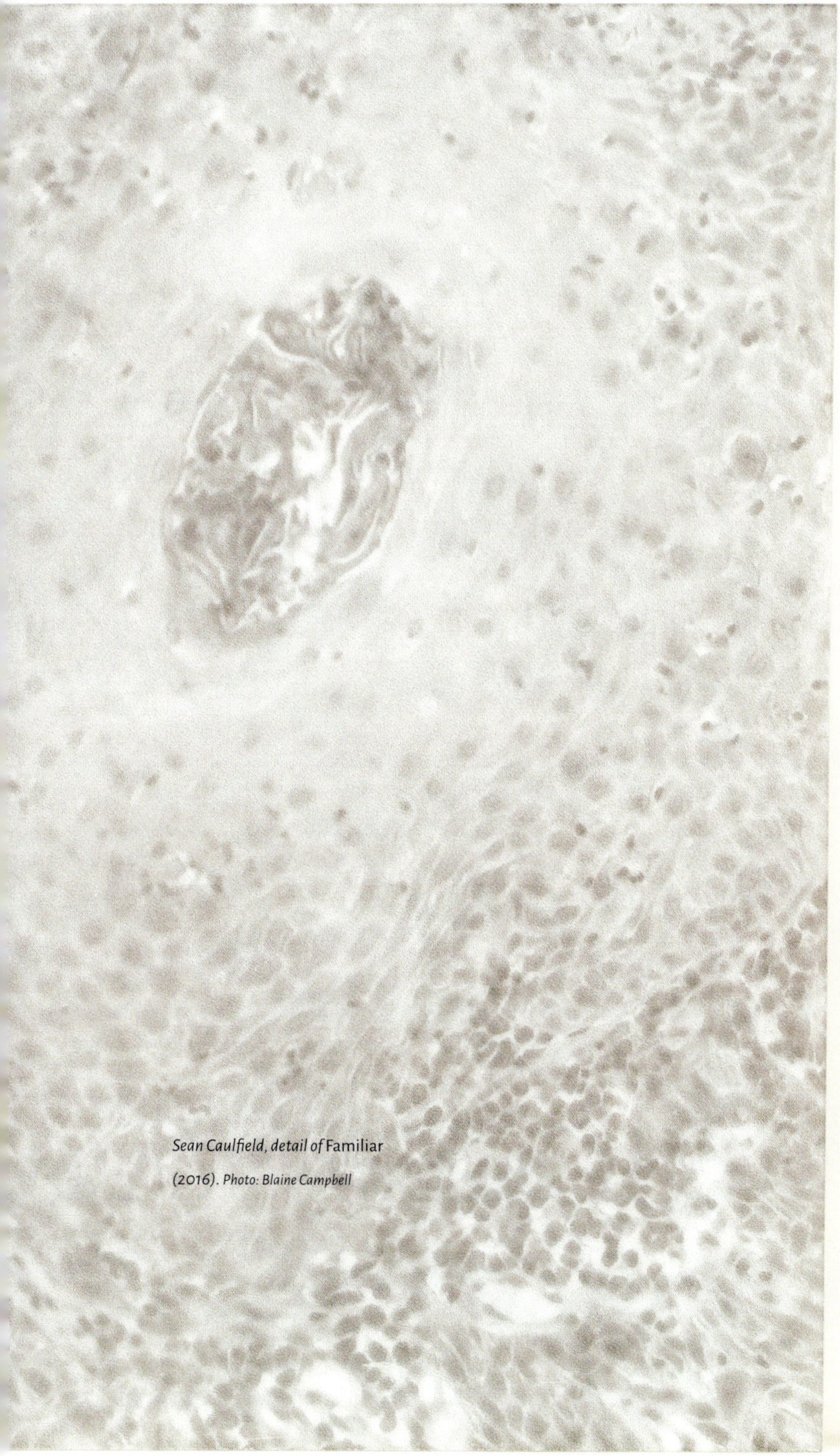

Sean Caulfield, detail of Familiar (2016). *Photo: Blaine Campbell*

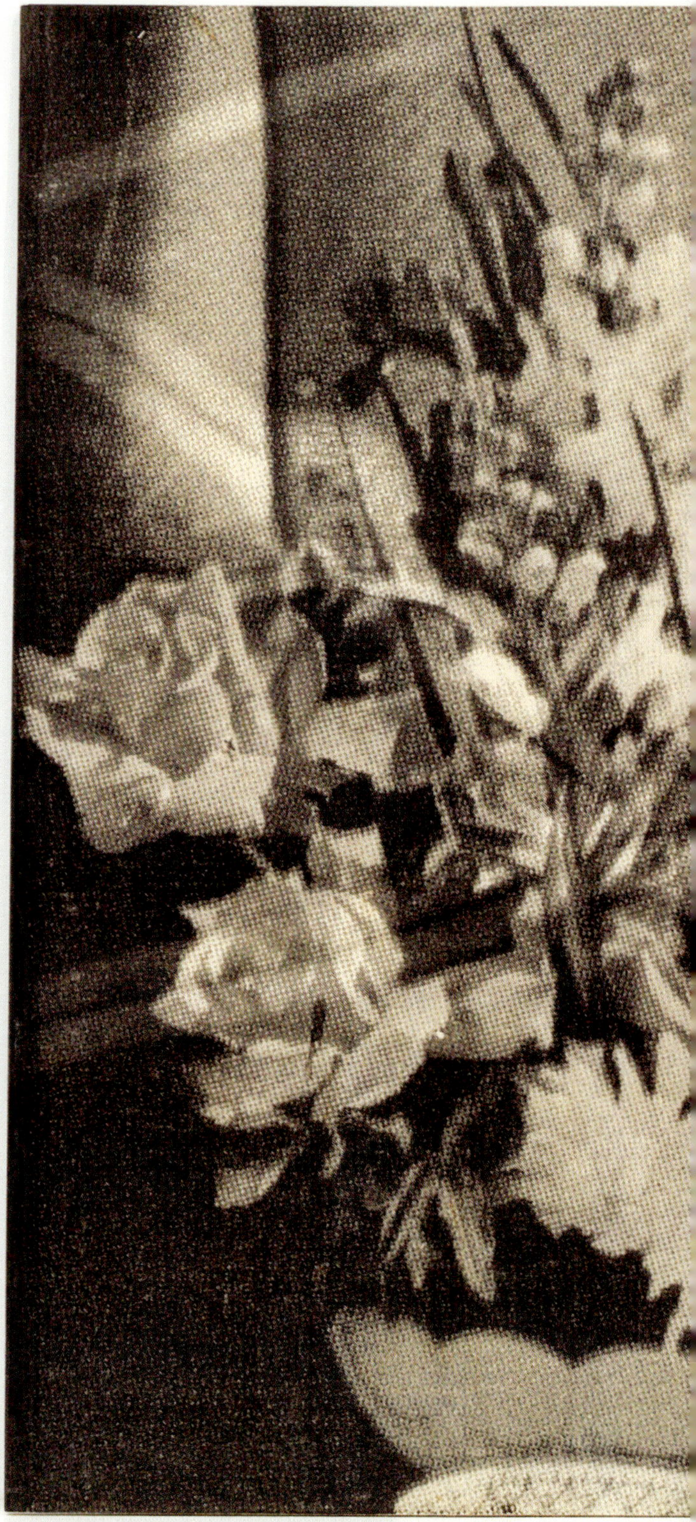

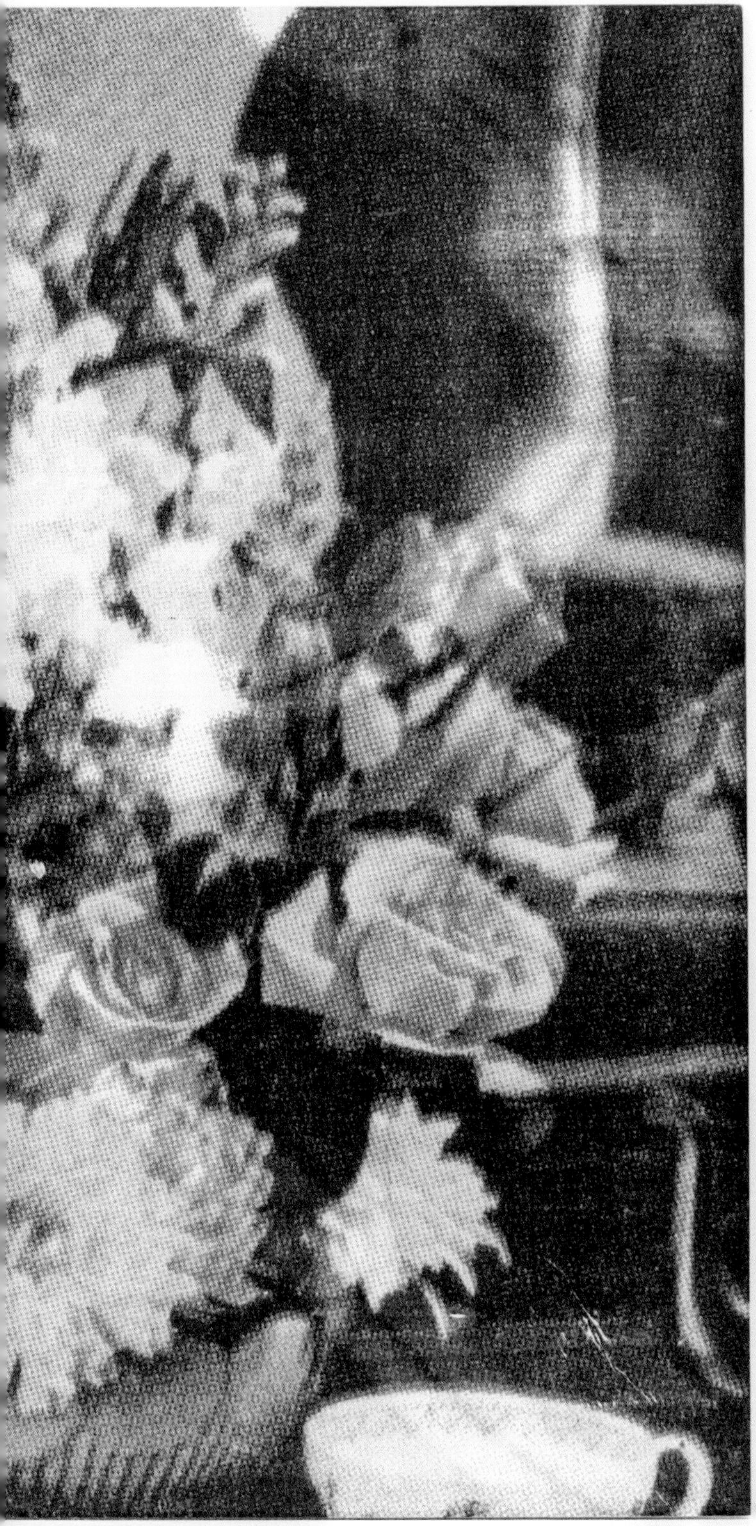

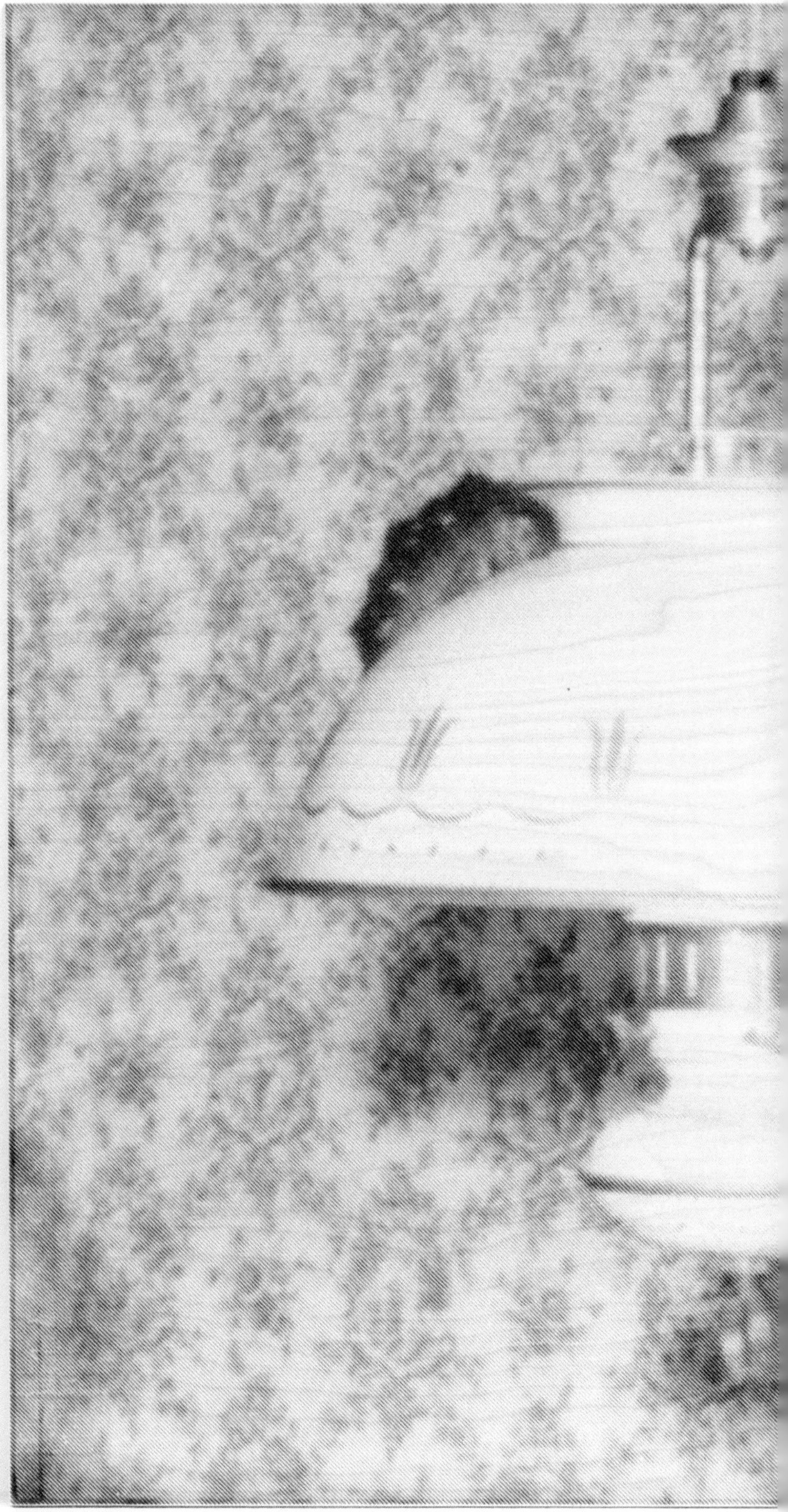

Ingrid Bachmann

When I speak the muscles
in my throat and mouth
have a memory of the
words spoken.

My ears retain an aural
memory of the words
heard.

What does it mean to lose one's voice? To lose the ability to laugh? To choose to be silent, or be silenced? These were some of the questions that arose for me through my participation in this project. People who have had a laryngectomy need to relearn how to speak. That process often involves multiple surgeries and years of physiotherapy and speech therapy. Even once speech has been relearned, the effort it takes can be arduous—and this doesn't even take into account the added effort of being understood. The impact of head and neck cancer on social interaction—ways of being together that most of us take for granted—is enormous. It makes interactions from the impersonal and mundane—conversations with cashiers or servers—to the personal and special—family dinners, nights out with friends—difficult, if not impossible.

Life after cancer can be good, but it is an altered life—and that needs to be acknowledged. This new life often includes a substantial physical alteration of the body that can profoundly affect an individual's sense of identity. There are also very real financial implications of illness, treatment, and recovery. I created my works in response to these observations.

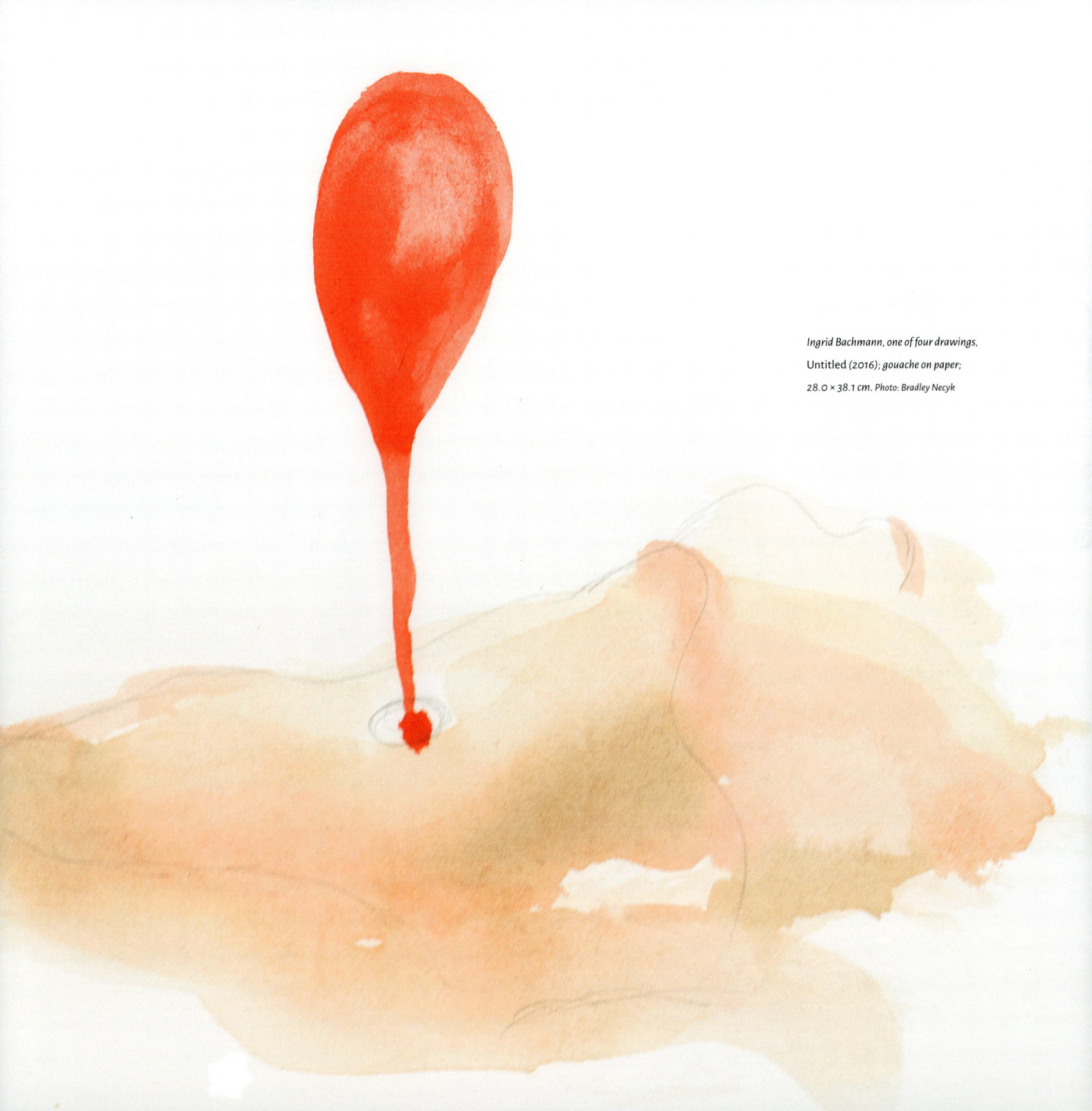

Ingrid Bachmann, one of four drawings, Untitled *(2016); gouache on paper;* 28.0 × 38.1 cm. *Photo: Bradley Necyk*

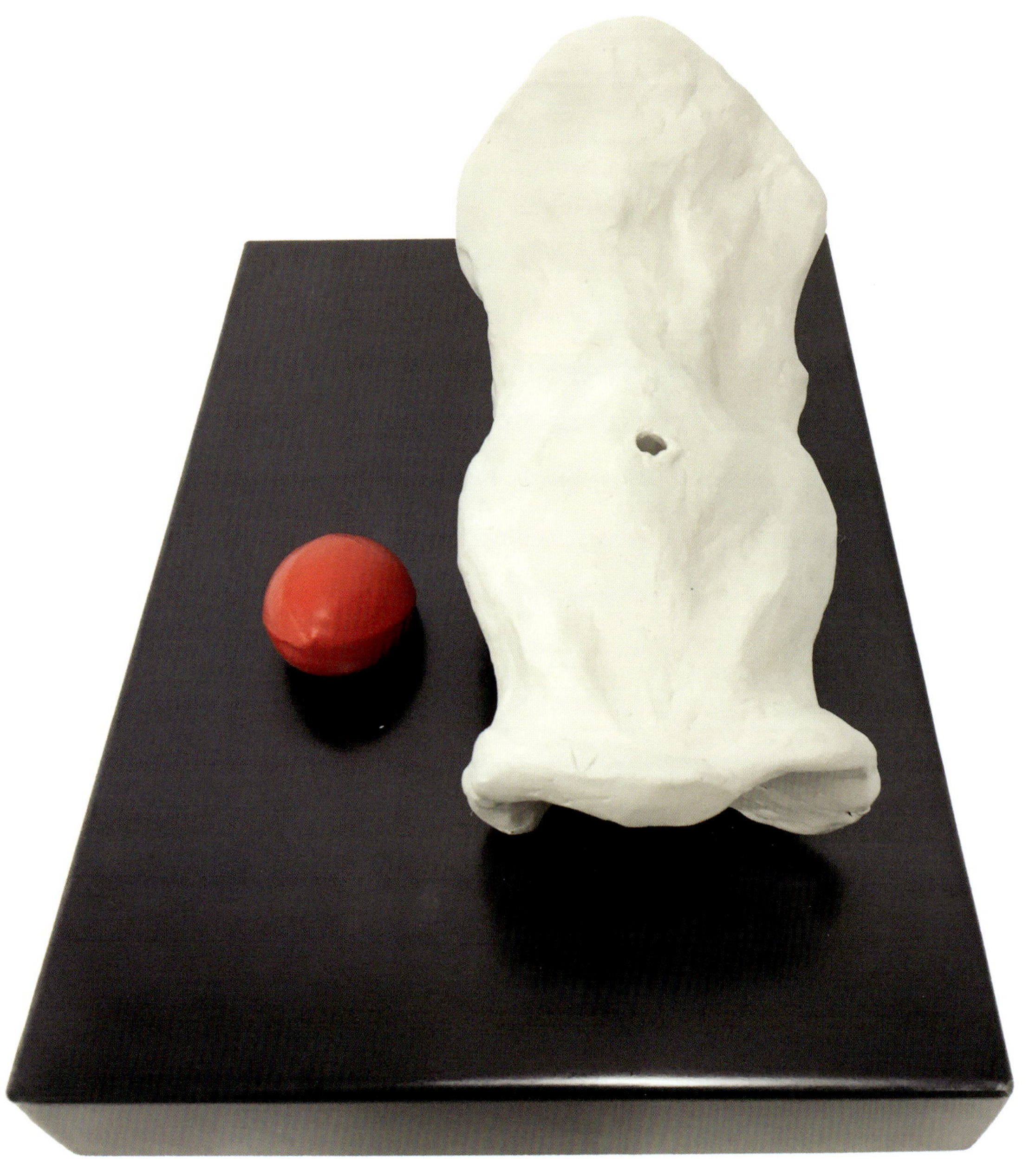

Ingrid Bachmann, Untitled (2016); *clay, red balloon; dimensions variable (support: 48.3 × 38.1 cm).*

Photo: Wojtek Gwiazda

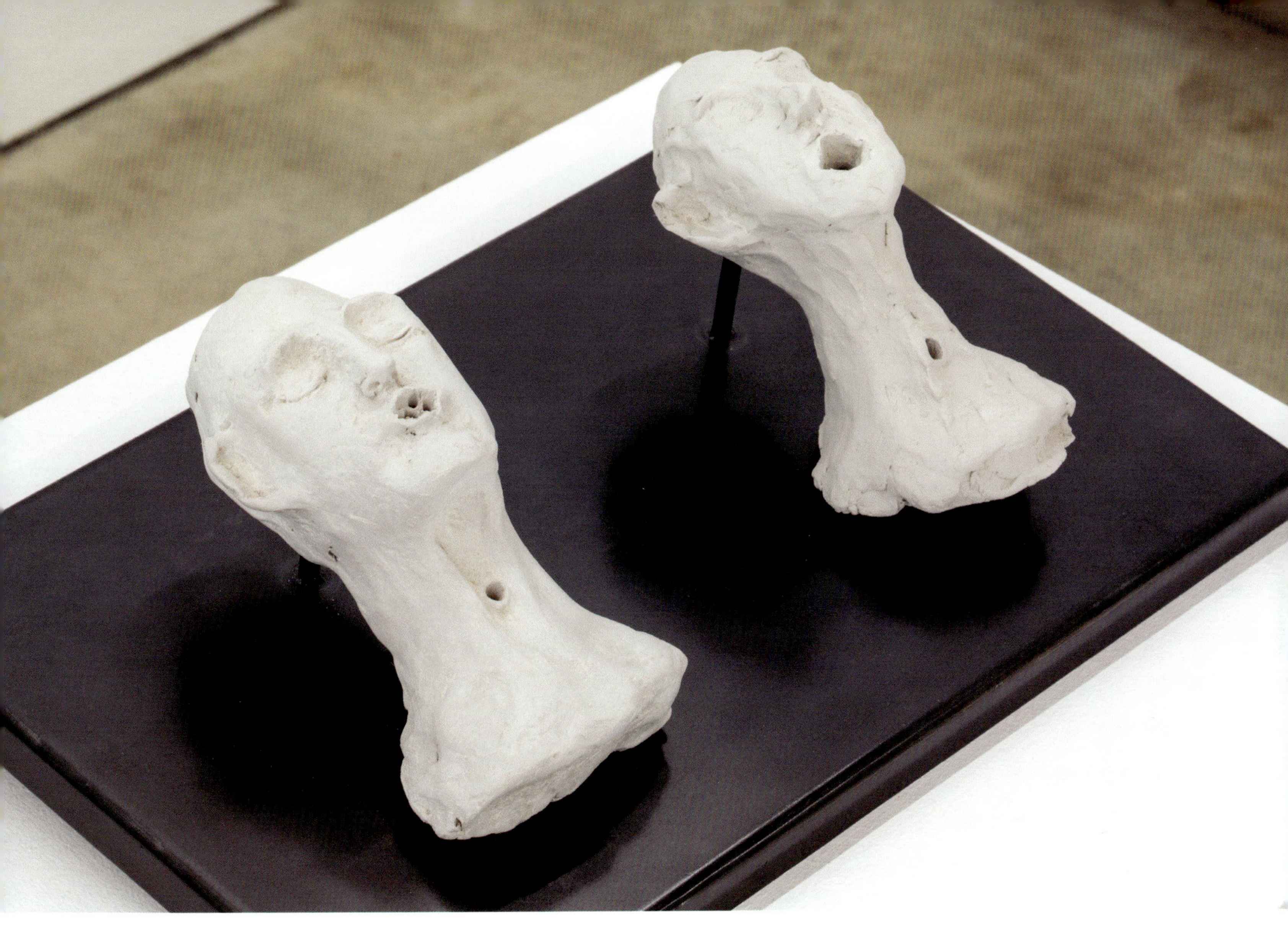

Ingrid Bachmann, Two Heads *(2016); clay and steel; 17.8 × 7.6 × 7.6 cm and 15.2 × 7.6 × 7.6 cm (support: 38.1 × 23.0 cm). Photo: Blaine Campbell*

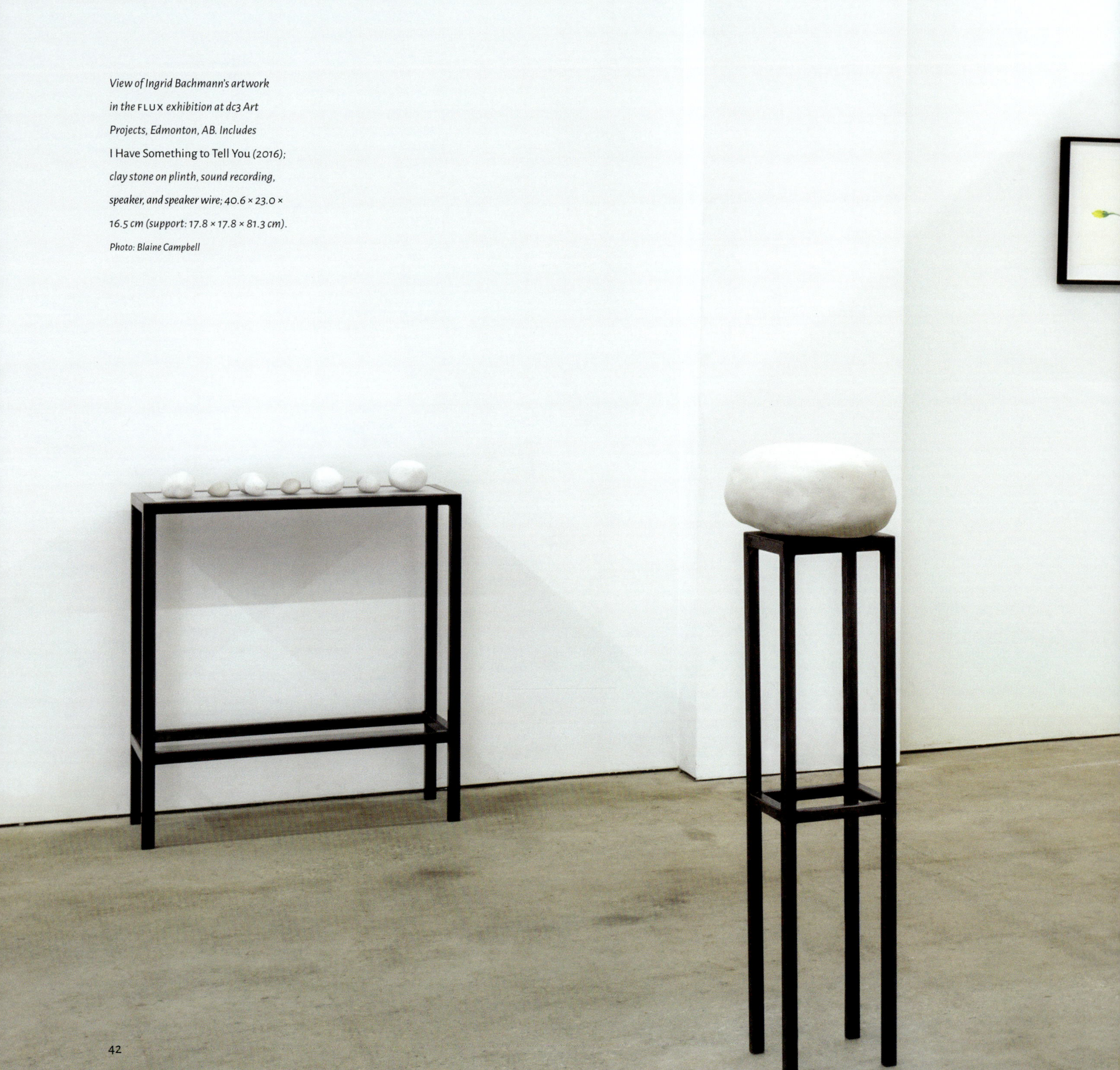

View of Ingrid Bachmann's artwork in the FLUX *exhibition at dc3 Art Projects, Edmonton, AB. Includes* I Have Something to Tell You (2016); *clay stone on plinth, sound recording, speaker, and speaker wire;* 40.6 × 23.0 × 16.5 cm *(support:* 17.8 × 17.8 × 81.3 cm*).*
Photo: Blaine Campbell

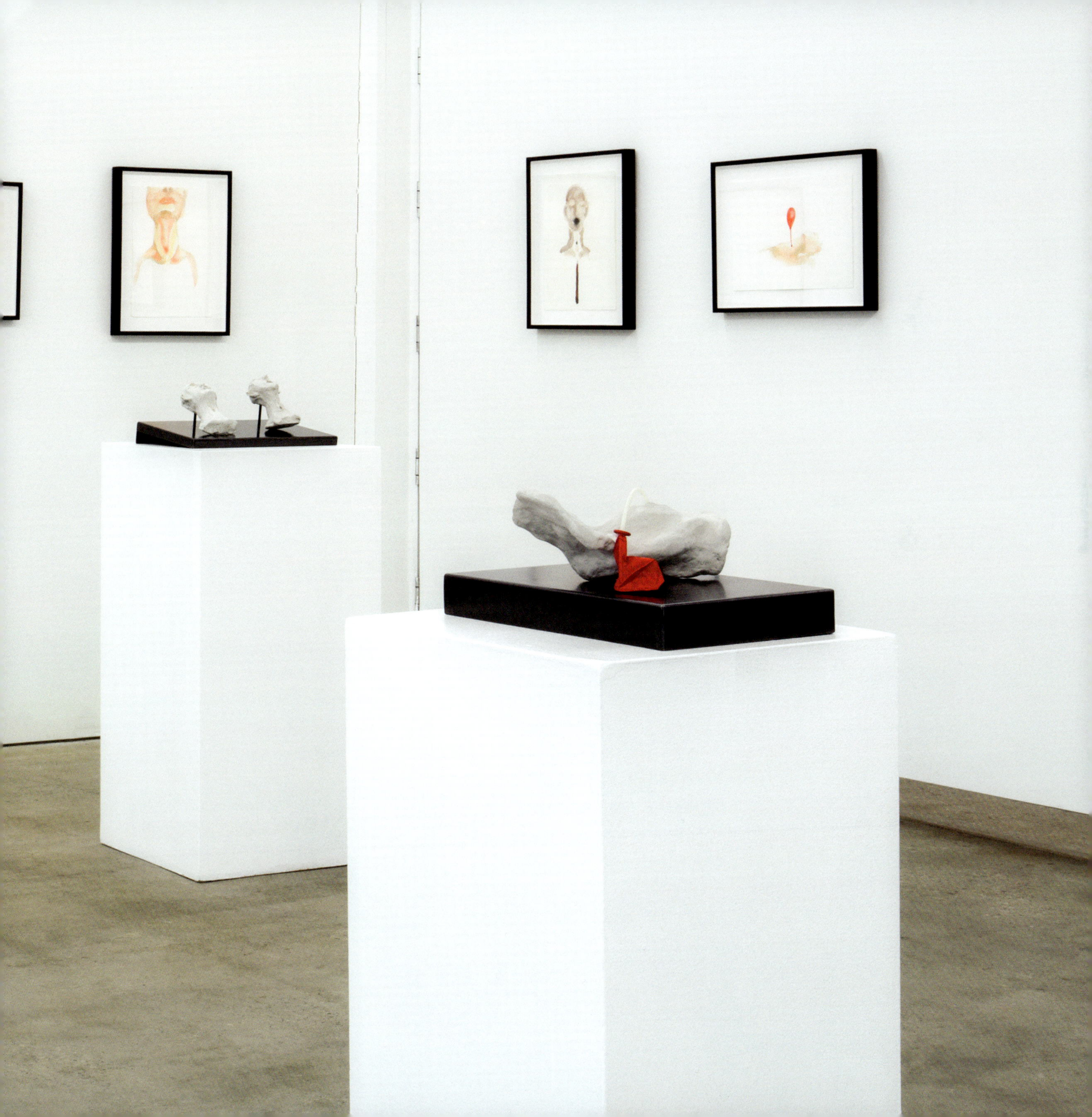

Bahaa Harmouche

When Design Meets Real Life

In October 2015, while completing my graduate degree in visual communication design, I became involved in the "see me, hear me, heal me" project. After agreeing to design various project identification materials, I was invited to participate in a two-day workshop facilitated by David Diamond, Artistic Director, Theatre for Living (Vancouver, BC). The workshop had been organized to introduce a collaborative research-creation inquiry process for the project. The workshop involved patients and their family members, as well as clinicians and health researchers. I imagined that I would simply learn a bit more about the overall project, and then go back to my design work. Little did I know, this workshop would change both my approach to design and my life.

At the time, I was reading about slow design, a method of design developed by Carolyn F. Strauss and Alastair Fuad-Luke[1] that is directed to developing "appropriately tailored" solutions for promoting the well-being of individuals and overall society. Similar to other "slow" movements (slow food, slow medicine, and the like), Strauss and Fuad-Luke emphasize a balanced approach to design informed by six principles: Reveal, Expand, Reflect, Engage, Participate, and Evolve. These principles are meant to guide designers in their approach and allow them to immerse themselves, through different lenses, in the design process, making way for a journey of self-discovery while redefining the core of design.

I have experienced slow design as a process of taking time to holistically connect with the subject I am working with. Intuition always plays a big part in the development of design solutions. However, intuition must be followed up with more intentional thought, and I have discovered that further reflection can promote deeper understanding of and connection to my subject. This, in turn, can lead to a myriad of other design possibilities. The "see me, hear me, heal me" project introduced me to new

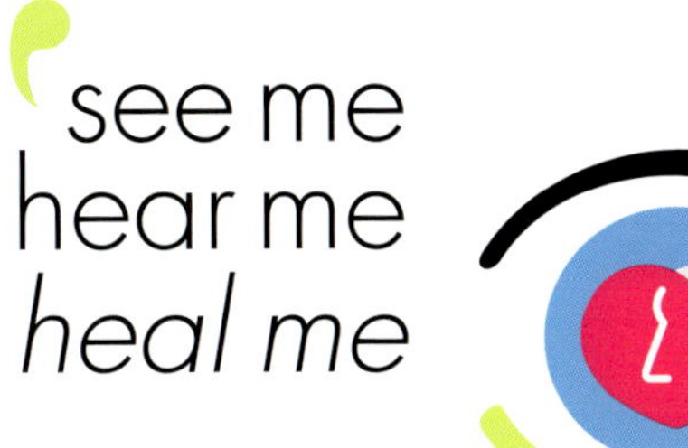

Bahaa Harmouche, designer, "see me, hear me, heal me" project logo (2015).

modes of reflection, and to the value of experiential, collaborative, and relational inquiry within the context of a focused yet open-ended workshop setting.

I experienced the workshop as profoundly moving and eye opening. The experiences and stories shared by patients recovering from head and neck cancer highlighted their struggle to reintegrate into society and to be heard. The workshop provided a setting in which senses and emotions mixed together. Through my participation, I became more than just a designer in the room; I was able to connect with the experience of others on a human level, outside of the confines of a specific role. Over the course of two short days, my involvement in the project transformed from being simply focused on conceptualizing visual identification materials for the project to a personal involvement in a deeper, more synergistic, human-centred process that has touched my soul and changed me forever.

The workshop also had a great impact on my design process. I experienced my work shifting from generic concepts to more meaningful representations. I appropriated a dominant visual that stayed with me after the workshop—the stoma, or opening, created in the front of the neck that allowed patients who had their voice boxes surgically removed to breathe. I incorporated this dominant visual in my logo design by representing it as a keyhole, connoting a deep space that holds both pain and power at the same time. There is the painful recollection of multiple surgical interventions that will always be part of the life of a patient who has had head and neck cancer. The shape also denotes, however, the vibrant presence and voice of patients who sometimes struggle to be heard as they work to make others aware and mindful of their presence. The keyhole shape symbolizes the beginning of connection and a discourse that can both promote a sense of belonging and bring communities together. The bright colours convey the powerful energy and love of life that the cancer patients projected to everyone involved in the "see me, hear me, heal me" project.

Any design problem that involves or affects people must begin by fully understanding and valuing the needs of those involved, and by placing their experience and well-being at the centre of the research. The well-being of individuals is directly connected to the well-being of the community and the natural environment in which they live. Recognizing this, and addressing design issues in a holistic manner, extends the question of design method beyond aesthetic, form, and utility concerns to an approach that incorporates a humanistic, soulful sensitivity that can bring a holistic essence to any design.[2]

Involving designers in collaborative projects focused on health and social issues can help effect a paradigm shift in industrial design, shifting it from a discipline that focuses on aesthetic and trend solutions to one that involves creatively engaging with pragmatic, critical, and human-centred dimensions of design. Training designers to think empathically will create a new generation of designers who hold high ethical standards and commit to contributing to the well-being of others and the world we in which we live.[3] The function of design will transform to include the role of social protector, which, in my opinion, is the holistic ideal to which all designers should aspire, and tirelessly work to achieve.

NOTES

1. Strauss, C.F. & Fuad-Luke, A. (2008). *The slow design principles: A new interrogative and reflexive tool for design and research practice*. Paper presented at the Changing the Change: Design Visions, Proposals, and Tools Conference, Turin, Italy. Retrieved from https://www.slowlab.net/RESOURCES/Resources-PUBLICATIONS-Slow-reading-s.
2. Fuad-Luke, A. (2007). *Reflection, consciousness, progress: Creatively slow designing the present*. Paper presented at the Reflections on Creativity: Exploring the Role of Theory in Creative Practices Conference, University of Dundee, Scotland. Retrieved from https://www.slowlab.net/RESOURCES/Resources-PUBLICATIONS-Slow-reading-s.
3. Findeli, A. (2001). Rethinking design education for the 21st century: Theoretical, methodological, and ethical discussion. *Design Issues*, 17(1), 5–17. https://www.jstor.org/stable/1511905.

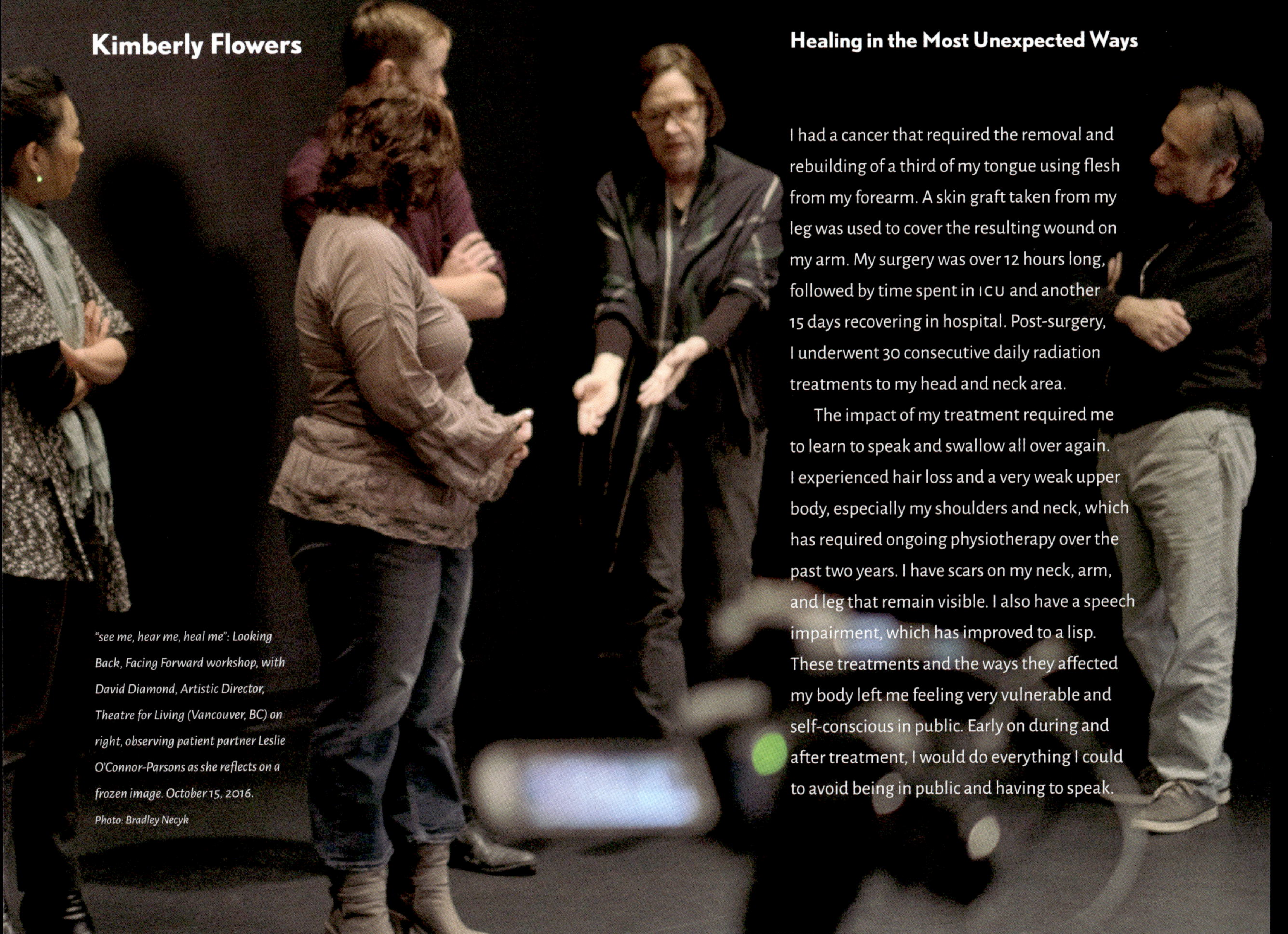

Kimberly Flowers

Healing in the Most Unexpected Ways

I had a cancer that required the removal and rebuilding of a third of my tongue using flesh from my forearm. A skin graft taken from my leg was used to cover the resulting wound on my arm. My surgery was over 12 hours long, followed by time spent in ICU and another 15 days recovering in hospital. Post-surgery, I underwent 30 consecutive daily radiation treatments to my head and neck area.

The impact of my treatment required me to learn to speak and swallow all over again. I experienced hair loss and a very weak upper body, especially my shoulders and neck, which has required ongoing physiotherapy over the past two years. I have scars on my neck, arm, and leg that remain visible. I also have a speech impairment, which has improved to a lisp. These treatments and the ways they affected my body left me feeling very vulnerable and self-conscious in public. Early on during and after treatment, I would do everything I could to avoid being in public and having to speak.

"see me, hear me, heal me": Looking Back, Facing Forward workshop, with David Diamond, Artistic Director, Theatre for Living (Vancouver, BC) on right, observing patient partner Leslie O'Connor-Parsons as she reflects on a frozen image. October 15, 2016.

Photo: Bradley Necyk

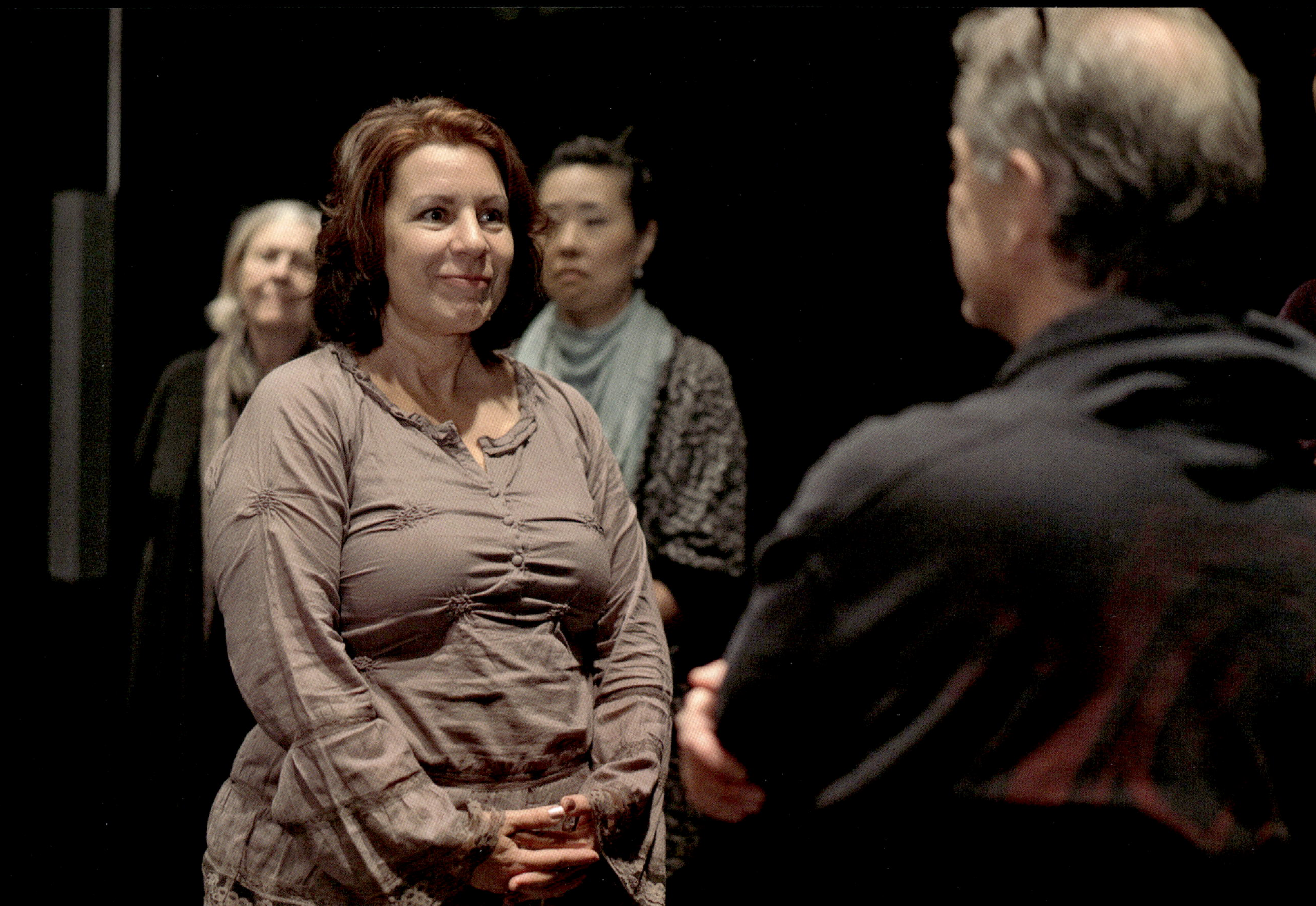

When I did go out or have a visitor, I covered myself with scarves and long-sleeved clothes and spoke very little.

I have been involved as a patient partner from the outset of the "see me, hear me, heal me" project. I participated in an initial interview and shortly thereafter was invited to participate in the introductory image theatre workshop. I was apprehensive about attending a workshop with complete strangers and participating in theatre exercises, but overcame my hesitancy when the process was described to me and I was given the freedom to participate as little or as much as I felt comfortable.

I appreciated the safety of the process and began to truly feel part of the research team. It was very liberating for me to have a group of people patiently take time to listen to and *"see me, hear me, heal me" Looking Back, Facing Forward workshop with patient partner Kimberly Flowers facing facilitator David Diamond. October 15, 2016.* Photo: *Bradley Necyk*

understand what I was saying. The simple act of being listened to without judgement boosted my confidence. I was also invited to sit in on the artists' planning session that immediately followed the image theatre workshop. Not only did this make me feel valued, but it helped me to understand the creative process from the artists' perspective.

About six months later, we gathered together again, and the artists presented their initial art pieces. I gained further insight into their creative process and how they incorporated patient experiences such as my own into their artworks. What was even more surprising to me was that these artists wanted our feedback as patients! They asked, Did their work clearly convey the messages they hoped to communicate? How much graphic detail should be included? How should the exhibition be set up and presented? By being consulted, I felt that I was heard and understood.

I left that session that day having to emotionally and psychologically process my reaction to the pieces the artists presented. I felt it provoked me—in a healthy way—to deal with the trauma of my cancer experience. I also had a sense of awe that these complete strangers could hear my experience as a patient and present it in a tangible, accurate way.

Later that fall, we again gathered in a workshop session led by David Diamond, Artistic Director, Theatre for Living (Vancouver, BC), and reflected on our journey to that point using the language of image theatre. It was amazing how far we had all come. I realized that I no longer felt like a patient, but instead identified more so as a patient advocate.

Sometimes healing comes in the most unexpected ways. Is it possible for holistic healing to be a meaningful addition to modern medicine? Yes, I believe it is.

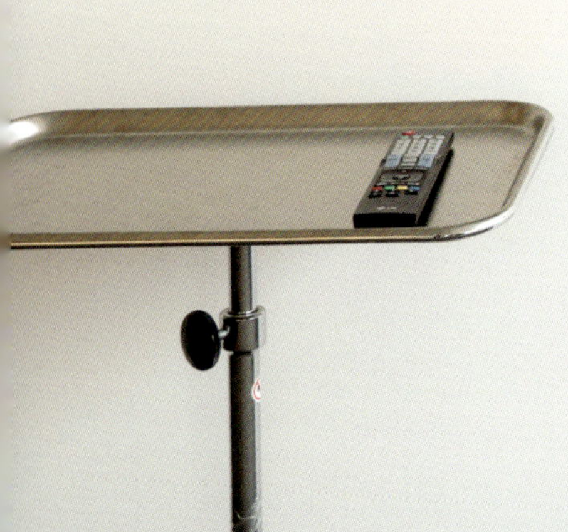

Still image of Bernie Krewski, patient partner, in Kyle Terrence's "see me, hear me, heal me" Video Documentation (2016) installed in the FLUX *exhibition entryway at dc3 Art Projects, Edmonton, AB.* Photo: Bradley Necyk

Kyle Terrence

"see me, hear me, heal me"
Video Documentation

I was asked to come in part way through the "see me, hear me, heal me" project as a documentarian. I had not been present for the first workshop; however, at the first meeting that I was able to attend, I noticed that there were already nuanced connections in the group dynamic. As I watched clinicians, patients, artists, and family members exchange pleasantries, I quickly realized that this would become the main lens through which I would observe this project: the smaller moments of contact between the participants during workshops, meetings, and critiques. I wanted to capture these, recognizing that the success of the overall project stemmed from these moments of connection.

I view the strength of this project as an effort to bridge the gap between the disparate experiences of a variety of people through other forms of knowing. My unique position as documentarian afforded me the opportunity to observe the larger process as an oscillation between various voices. Everyone in the group experienced anxiety in some form, sometimes during challenging, uncomfortable moments in workshops, or while sharing difficult stories of illness, or in vulnerable occasions when sharing artworks that had been inspired by another person's experiences.

As the baton was passed back and forth, I could see many of these anxieties dissolve into trust and new forms of understanding. The most profound moment for me was the moment I realized that the project was not building toward the development of a more sympathetic understanding of the patient experience in particular; rather, it was building toward a multilayered experience of empathy-building among all of the participants, both patient partners and other collaborators.

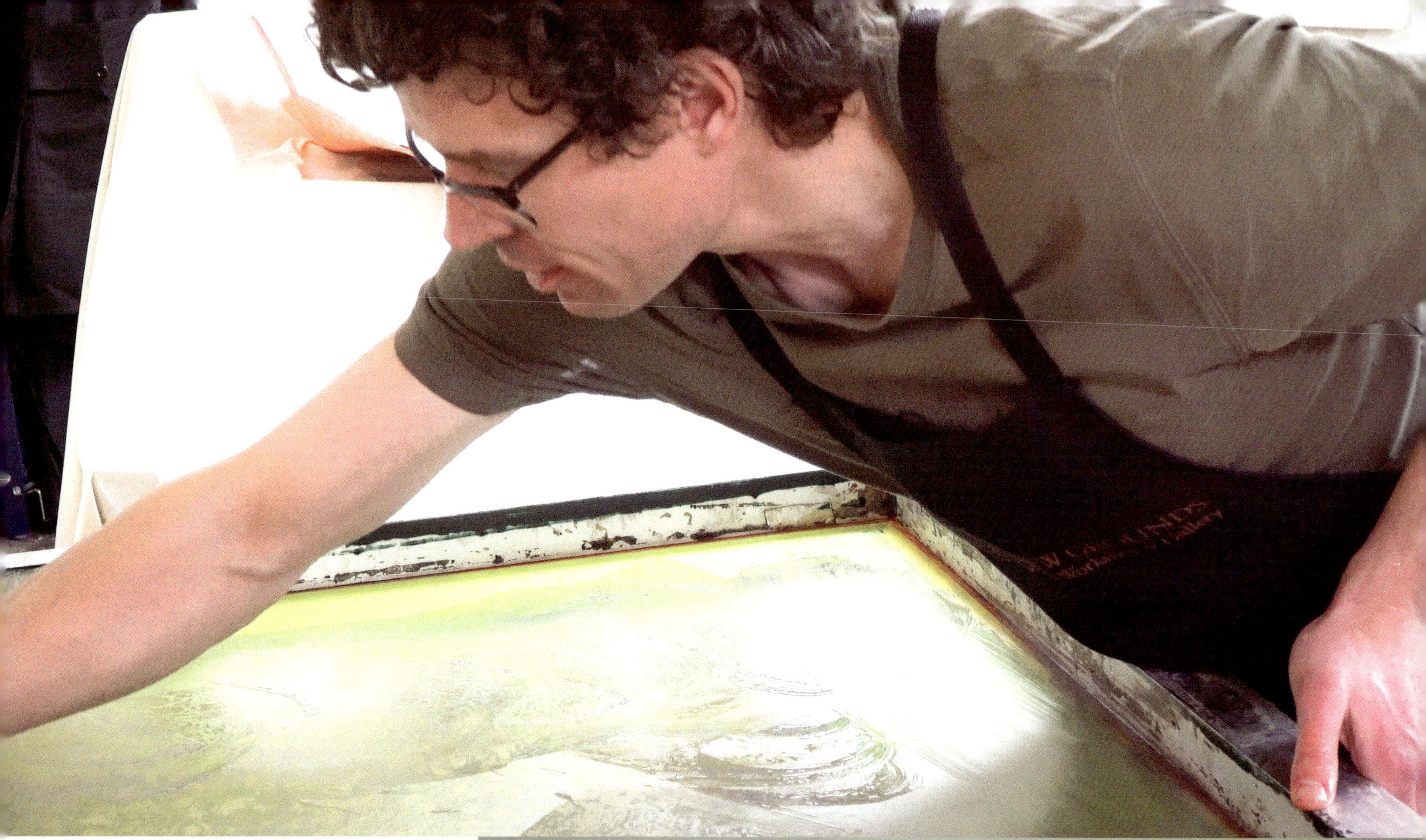

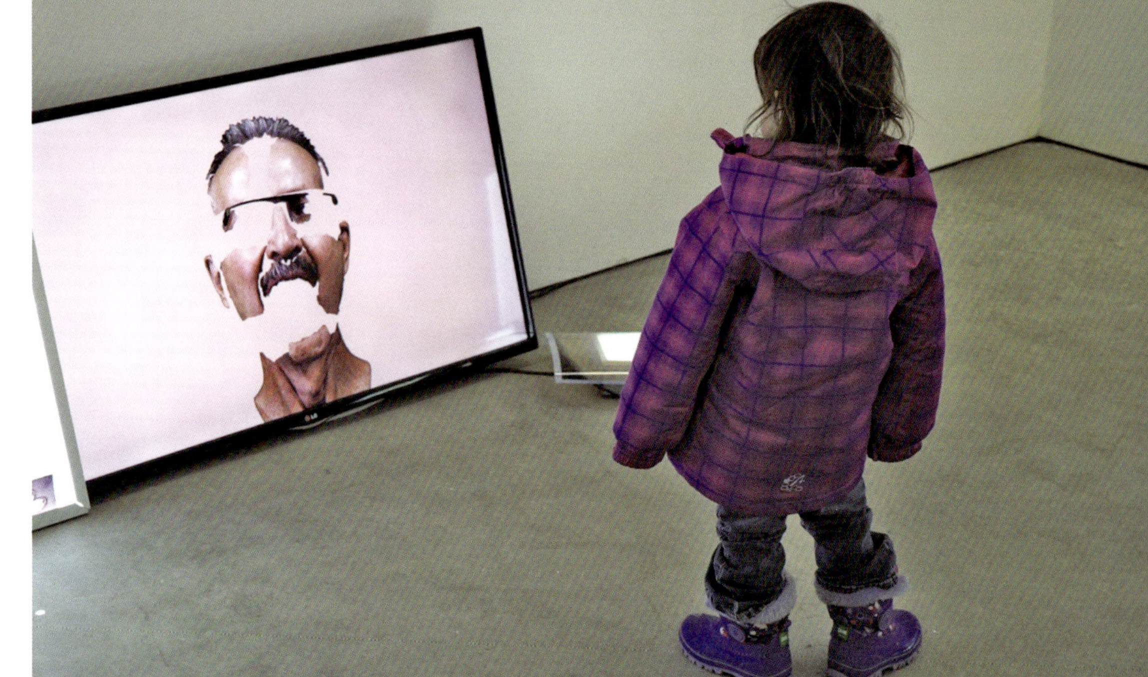

(top) Still image of artist participant Sean Caulfield in Kyle Terrence's "see me, hear me, heal me" Video Documentation (2016).

Photo: Kyle Terrence

(bottom) Still image of young exhibition visitor viewing Bradley Necyk's Waiting Room *(2016) in Kyle Terrence's "see me, hear me, heal me" Video Documentation (2016).*

Photo: Kyle Terrence

PAMELA BRETT-MACLEAN &
MINN N. YOON

Afterword
The "see me, hear me, heal me" Project as Research-Creation for Social Change

Founded on a commitment to meaningful engagement, our approach to research-creation involved a range of components directed to realizing generative outcomes and catalyzing change.[1] We began by setting a central, bold, and ambitious goal: We aimed to change the world.

We have directed our efforts to unmasking the hidden face of head and neck cancer by engaging diverse audiences in taking in, and responding to visually gripping portrayals of the experience of head and neck cancer. By doing so, we hope to facilitate understanding and catalyze support for patients as they undergo treatment and recovery, both within Canada and around the world.

An important first step was to engage people affected by head and neck cancer as part of the research-creation process. The "see me, hear me, heal me" project has involved ongoing collaboration among patients, family members, artists, clinicians, and health researchers. This dynamic, collaborative structure fostered multiple early connections, which strengthened our collective commitment to realizing shared project objectives.

We worked to support the development of team-based, relational capacities, and attended to the *process* of engagement, recognizing this to be integral to realizing our ambitious goals and objectives. As has been noted by several contributors, we engaged David Diamond, Artistic Director of Theatre for Living (Vancouver, BC) early on to facilitate relationship-building among all participants. This early event solidified our commitment to the project, by orienting us to the possibilities and promise of our collaborative venture. It offered a way for all of us, and especially our patient partners, to engage on a more equal footing from the very beginning. It also contributed to our commitment to ensuring opportunities for ongoing connection and dialogue. This commitment was reinforced over the course of the project as we engaged with each other in various ways. The breadth of perspectives and experiences across the team contributed to a guiding, collective intelligence that has helped to ensure impactful project outcomes in the form of events and activities that support meaningful connections and relationships. Outcomes, which continue to unfold, include new projects inspired by the "see me, hear me, heal me" project.

Artistic exhibitions offer a particularly effective means for expressive communication that can heighten engagement by evoking emotional responses. These imaginative spaces provide an opportunity for "seeing connections" and developing embodied understandings, resulting in greater capacity for personal and cultural creativity than that afforded by Cartesian-based, rational calculation. Located within a physical space, with artworks situated just so, art exhibitions serve to encourage reflection and dialogue. John Shotter argues that experiences such as these offer a particular kind of telling that leads to affective responses or artistic perception that can point to better ways of going forward. Building on the ideas of William James, Ludwig Wittgenstein, and others, Shotter suggests that "although all is in flux, we can still find the guidance we need for our own thinking within the dynamics of our own movements of feeling."[2]

From the very beginning of the "see me, hear me, heal me" project, we have followed processes that have shaped and reshaped us. We have organized, and continue to organize, events that have promoted both casual discussion and more formal dialogue and deliberation. These events have offered a means of engagement that has supported new beginnings and ongoing "relational becomings." These processes have both transformed us and created openings for more positive future possibilities—not only for those who have been impacted by head and neck cancer, but also, we hope, for the larger world.

NOTE

1. Core aspects and principles informing our aesthetic, relational research approach are outlined in in Yoon, M.N., & Brett-MacLean, P. (in press). Living stories: An arts-based, relational research framework directed to transformative change in healthcare. In D. Dole, E. Raboin, P. Thomas, et al. (Eds.), *Social Construction in Action: The Taos Institute's Silver Jubilee*. Chagrin Falls, OH: Taos Institute Publications.
2. Shotter, J. (2016). *Speaking, actually: Towards a new "fluid" common-sense understanding of relational becomings.* Farnhill, UK: Everything is Connected Press. Shotter lists four stages typically associated with decision-making processes: 1) perceive a situation, 2) consider possible courses of action, 3) identify a "best" course of action (often, closely aligned with one's own interests), and 4) follow the selected course, rationalizing the decision in relation to factors that support it (178). Given that things coming into being are always indeterminant and open to many possibilities, Shotter suggests that we "shift our focus from step three (3)—*arriving at after-the-fact conclusions as a result of calculational reasoning*—to exploring the nature of the *before-the-fact processes* involved in *coming to a specific perception* of WHAT the situation, that we are 'in', *is like*, to examine step one (1), our perception of the situation we are in" (180, italics and all capitals text in original). He maintains that by immersing ourselves "in the 'happening' of those 'in-the-moment' meanings...[a] holistic unity, that will enlarge the array of human possibilities available to us, will emerge" (181).

MINN N. YOON &
PAMELA BRETT-MACLEAN

Project Timeline

2015

June

- Minn first meets with Jane at Starbucks. Development of visual approaches to research around patient experiences of head and neck cancer commences.
- The "see me, hear me, heal me" project is conceptualized. Steps are taken to realize this vision, including meeting with potential collaborators, submitting funding proposals, and a research ethics application.

September

- University of Alberta Health Research Ethics Board approves the "Head and Neck Cancer Illness Experiences" protocol (PRO00060143). Amendments to the protocol are submitted throughout the project to cover new activities that develop as the project evolves.

October

- The "see me, hear me, heal me" team receives grant funding from Alberta Innovates (Community Engagement and Conference Grant) and the Kule Institute for Advanced Studies, University of Alberta (Kule Research Team Grant).
- Qualitative research for the "see me, hear me, heal me" project begins. Interviews are conducted and videotaped with patient participants and family members. Interviews continue until the end of September 2016.
- The "see me, hear me, heal me": Introductory Workshop is held, focused on the theme "Transforming Understandings of Patients' Experiences of Head and Neck Cancer." The workshop spans two days.

  Day 1: evening reception / networking event directed to introduction and relationship building; formal welcome and opening remarks (Minn N. Yoon); presentation on contemporary art (Sean Caulfield); poster viewing (including posters focused on the experience of head and neck cancer with excerpts from interview transcripts organized into five themes—food and eating, social life, appearance, communication, and resilience—and posters highlighting information about and artwork of the participating artists); introduction to image theatre work (David Diamond); closing remarks (Minn N. Yoon).

Day 2: relationship-building circle; image theatre exercises; "walk and talk with me" exercises involving one-on-one discussions between patients and artists; debriefing session; closing remarks (Minn N. Yoon); written reflections; optional meeting to discuss the next phase of the "see me, hear me, heal me" project.

- Tours of the Edmonton-based Institute for Reconstructive Sciences in Medicine (iRSM; www.ualberta.ca/reconstructive-medical-sciences), an internationally recognized institute focused on clinical care, research, education and training in reconstructive medicine and technology sciences take place both before and following the initial workshop.

November

- The "see me, hear me, heal me" project's brand identity and logo are developed.
- Exhibition space is secured at dc3 Art Projects (Edmonton, AB). Detailed exhibition planning begins. Lianne McTavish (exhibition curator) applies and receives funding for the *FLUX* exhibition from the Killam Research Fund, University of Alberta.

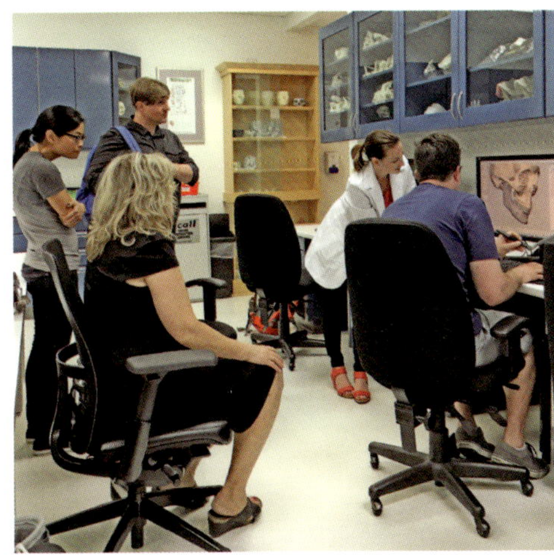

Artist participants on a tour of the Institute for Reconstructive Medicine, November 2, 2015, Edmonton, AB.

Photo: Minn N. Yoon

- As part of the artwork development process, ongoing contact is established between artists, patients, and family members until their next official meeting in July 2016. Researchers maintain communications with patients, family members, and artists, respond to inquiries, share updates and opportunities, and organize team meetings.

2016

July

- An additional tour of the iRSM is held for those unable to take part in the tours organized in the fall of 2015.
- An informal reception is held at FAB Gallery (University of Alberta) for patients, health care researchers, artists, friends, and colleagues prior to the "see me, hear me, heal me": Artists' Sharing Workshop.

- The "see me, hear me, heal me": Artists' Sharing Workshop is held at the University of Alberta. Artists share the ideas and preliminary work they have developed in relation to the project with patients, families, and other members of the project team. Patients and family members are invited to respond to the artists by giving feedback and sharing their reflections.
- Lianne McTavish organizes visits to artists' studios for patient partners and their family members. Visits are ongoing until October 2016.
- Artists remain in contact with patients and family members through 2016. Researchers remain in contact with patients, family members, and artists, ensuring ongoing, timely communication regarding various project developments, including planning related to the installation of the FLUX exhibition at dc3 Art Projects (Edmonton, AB) in January 2017.

August

- The "see me, hear me, heal me" project team is nominated by the University of Alberta for the prestigious Canadian Institutes for Health Research (CIHR) Gold Leaf Prize for Innovation: Patient Engagement. Team members prepare documents and gather letters in support of this nomination.

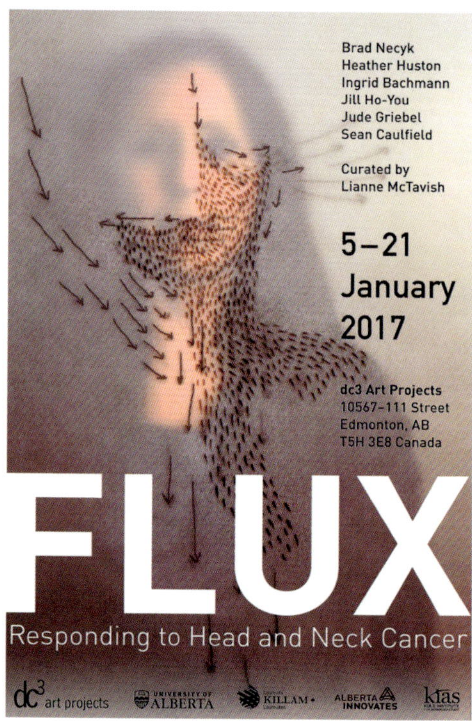

FLUX: Responding to Head and Neck Cancer *poster featuring artwork by Heather Huston for the dc3 Art Projects exhibition (January 2017), Edmonton, AB.* *Design: Bahaa Harmouche*

October

- The "see me, hear me, heal me": Looking Back, Facing Forward workshop is held at the University of Alberta. Facilitated by David Diamond, this half-day workshop offers an opportunity to pause and reflect on our journey to date through embodied, sculpted image-making.

2017

January

- The FLUX: *Responding to Head and Neck Cancer* exhibition is held at dc3 Art Projects (Edmonton, AB; www.dc3artprojects.com).

see me
hear me
heal me

Art that reveals hidden aspects of patient experiences with ***head and neck cancer***

June 22 - August 3, 2017

Opening Reception June 28 7-9pm

McMULLEN GALLERY

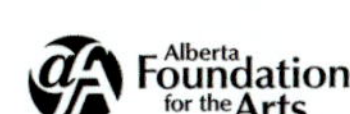

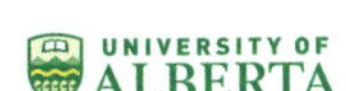

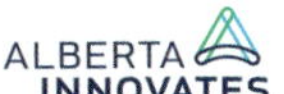

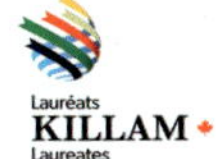

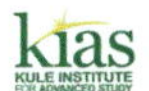

"see me, hear me, heal me" *poster featuring artwork by Ingrid Bachmann for the McMullen Gallery exhibition (June–August 2017), Edmonton, AB. Design: Tyler Sherard*

Over 300 people attend the opening reception on January 5.

- The exhibition attracts local, national, and international media coverage.
- Several events are organized in conjunction with the FLUX exhibition:

  January 12: A Science in the Cinema presentation of the documentary film *Life Itself* (about the life and death of Roger Ebert) is held, sponsored by the Faculty of Medicine & Dentistry at the University of Alberta and with post-screening respondents Drs. Vincent Biron and Jana Rieger.

  January 17: The Kule Institute for Advanced Study sponsors the Arts, Humanities, Social Sciences, Health, and Medicine edition of the Kule Connect Café.

  January 19: Reflections on FLUX, a community dialogue event organized with patient partners, participating artists, and other team members, is held.

- Throughout run, exhibition tours guided by patient partners and curator Lianne McTavish are organized for different health profession groups involving both educators and students.
- A total of 559 people view the exhibition over the course of its run, which concludes January 19.

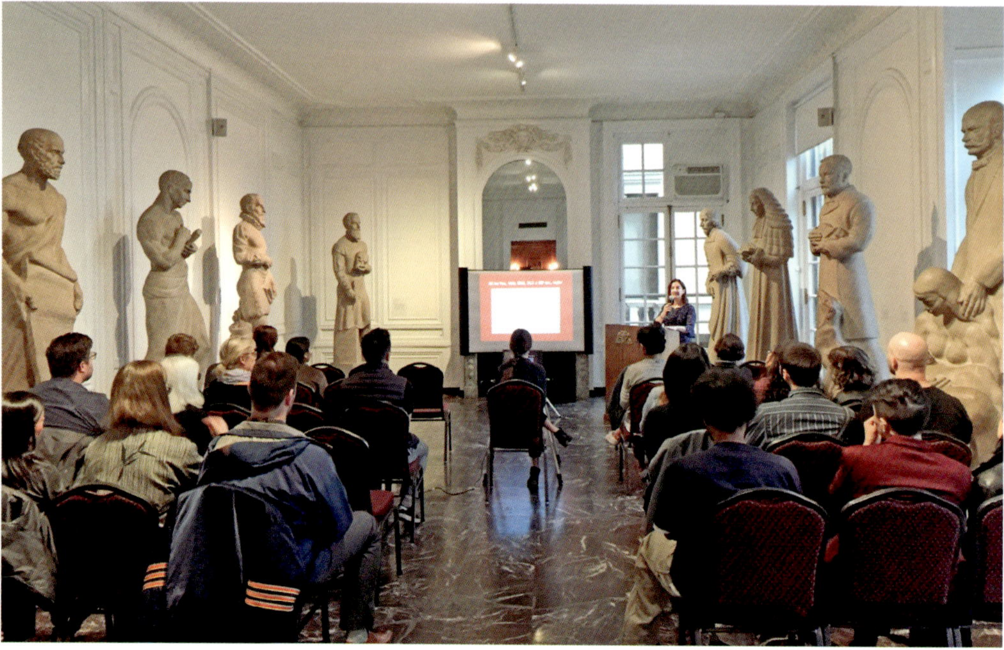

Lianne McTavish delivers a curatorial talk in the Hall of Immortals at the International Museum of Surgical Science as part of the FLUX *exhibition, Chicago, IL. May 18, 2018.*

Photo: Wojtek Gwiazda

February

- The dc3 Art Projects exhibition of *FLUX* is featured in *Canadian Art*.[1]

March

- The dc3 Art Projects exhibition of *FLUX* is featured in *The Lancet: Oncology*.[2]

June

- The "see me, hear me, heal me" project mounts an exhibition at the McMullen Gallery at the University of Alberta Hospital (Edmonton, AB; http://www.friendsofuah.org/mcmullen-gallery). Organized in conjunction with "The Works Art & Design Festival" (www.theworks.ab.ca), the exhibition features artwork created for the original *FLUX* exhibition.
- An opening reception and panel discussion held on June 28; patient-led tours take place over the run of the exhibition.
- 854 visitors attend over the course of the seven-week exhibition from June 22 to August 3.

2018

May

- The *FLUX*: *Responding to Head and Neck Cancer* exhibition is mounted at the International Museum of Surgical Science (IMSS; Chicago, IL; https://imss.org).

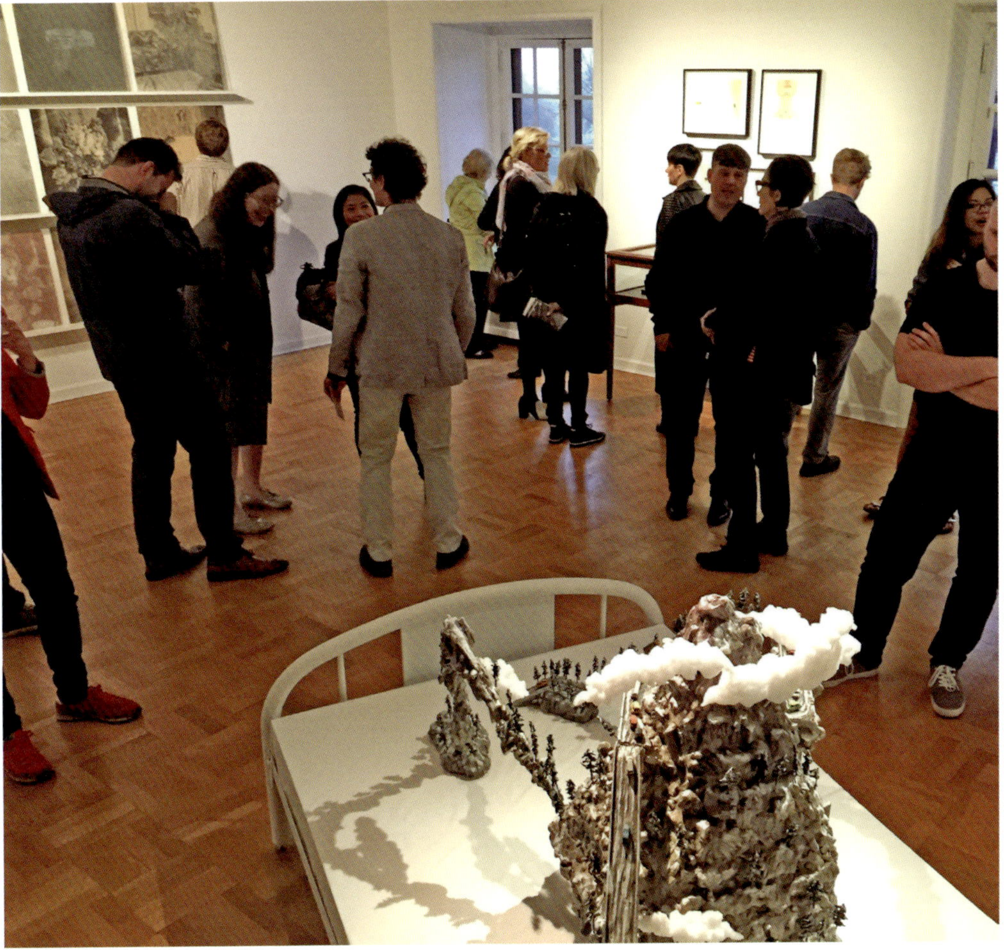

Visitors attending the opening of the FLUX *exhibition at the International Museum of Surgical Science, May 18, 2018, Chicago, IL.*
Photo: Wojtek Gwiazda

- Additional events are organized to promote the *FLUX* exhibition in Chicago.
  May 18: An opening reception and curator talk is given.
  May 19: The Undergoing *FLUX*: Art–Medicine Collaborative Praxis symposium is held.
- Throughout run: Specific educational events take place, such as a group of 70 neurosurgery precollege students from the University of Chicago attending to discuss the exhibition.
- A total of 8,447 visitors attend during the course of the exhibition, from May 18 to August 19.
- Funding to support patient partner travel is received from the Patient Engagement Platform, Alberta SPOR SUPPORT Unit; and the IRSM, University of Alberta.

2019

January

- The IMSS exhibition in Chicago, Illinois, is featured in the *Canadian Medical Association Journal*.[3]

September

- *Art–Medicine Collaborative Practice: Transforming the Experience of Head and Neck Cancer* is published by the University of Alberta Press.

Ongoing

- In addition published scholarly work and numerous presentations about the FLUX exhibition and the overall project that have been delivered to diverse audiences by contributors to this text, we continue to share our experience and insights with diverse audiences locally, nationally, and internationally. The "see me, hear me, heal me" team continues to respond to opportunities for exhibiting FLUX. Enquiries can be directed to Minn Yoon at minn.yoon@ualberta.ca or livingstories.ca/smhmhm.

NOTES

1. Pratt, A. (2017, February 8). Canadian artists take on cancer. *Canadian Art*. Retrieved from http://canadianart.ca/reviews/canadian-artists-take-cancer.
2. Holmes, B. (2017). See me, hear me, heal me. *The Lancet Oncology*, *18*(3), 296. http://dx.doi.org/10.1016/S1470-2045(17)30116-X.
3. McTavish, L. (2019). FLUX: Responding to head and neck cancer. *Canadian Medical Association Journal*, *191*(3), E80-E81. https://doi.org/10.1503/cmaj.180818.

Contributors

Ingrid Bachmann explores the complicated relationship between material and virtual realms, using redundant and new technologies in her generative and interactive artworks. An associate professor in the Studio Arts Department at Concordia University (Montreal, QC), Bachmann exhibits her work nationally and internationally. She is co-editor of *Material Matters* (YYZ Books, 1998, 1999, 2011) and has contributed essays to periodicals and anthologies, including *The Object of Labor* (MIT Press, 2007). A founding member of Hexagram: Institute for Research and Creation in the Media Arts, she is also director of the Institute of Everyday Life, art-ideas research lab. (www.ingridbachmann.com)

Pamela Brett-MacLean, associate professor in the Department of Psychiatry and director of the Arts & Humanities in Health & Medicine program in the Faculty of Medicine & Dentistry at the University of Alberta, is committed to fostering humanism in medicine through arts-based, reflective, relational approaches. She has widely presented on her work, and has authored numerous articles and texts, including *Keeping Reflection Fresh: A Practical Guide for Clinical Educators* (Kent State University Press, 2016), a book she co-edited with Allan Peterkin. She also collaborated with Peterkin and others to establish the Canadian Association for Health Humanities, which was founded in 2018.

Sean Caulfield, Centennial Professor in the Department of Art & Design at the University of Alberta, has exhibited his prints, drawings, and artist's books extensively throughout Canada, the United States, Europe, and Japan. Caulfield has received numerous grants and awards for his work including Social Science and Humanities Research Council dissemination and fine arts creation grants (Canada), and the Triennial Prize at the 2nd Bangkok Triennial International Print and Drawing Exhibition (Thailand). Caulfield's work is in various public and private collections including Harvard University (USA); Fitzwilliam Museum, Cambridge (UK); and Blanton Museum of Art, University of Texas (USA). (www.seancaulfield.ca)

Kimberly Flowers has lived with head and neck cancer for three years. Flowers serves as an informal patient mentor with the Head and Neck Cancer Support Group at the University of Alberta Hospital in Edmonton, Alberta. She participates in numerous clinical trials and studies and is a member of the Institute for Reconstructive Science and Medicine (iRSM) patient advisory group. She also serves as the president of the Head and Neck Cancer Support Society (https://head-way.org). These initiatives empower her as she continues to live with the devastating, day-to-day reality of head and neck cancer. Among these activities, her involvement as a patient collaborator in the "see me, hear me, heal me" project holds a special place in her healing journey.

Jude Griebel explores themes of psychological unease and transformation in his sculptural work. Depicting bodies in various states of composition, his work examines abstract notions such as growth, consumption, and mortality through metaphorical and experiential avenues. His work has been exhibited nationally and internationally. A 2015 artist in residence at Halle 14 Centre for Contemporary Art, Leipzig (Germany), Griebel was also awarded the inaugural Alberta Foundation for the Arts residency at the International Studio and Curatorial Program in Brooklyn (USA). In addition to other funding awards, he is a three-time recipient of the Elizabeth Greenshields Foundation grant for international emerging artists. (www.judegriebel.com)

Bahaa Harmouche completed his Master of Design degree in the Department of Art & Design at the University of Alberta in 2017, after having spent 13 years working in the advertising industry in the Middle East and North Africa. His graduate studies focused on understanding the value of visual communication in relation to diverse sociocultural issues, in particular the representation of HIV/AIDS across regions, class, age, and sexual orientation. (www.bharmouche.com)

Jill Ho-You is assistant professor at the Alberta University of the Arts. Her practice examines the parallels between the landscape, built environment, and the human body. Her drawings, prints, and installations have been exhibited nationally and internationally, including solo exhibitions at SNAP Gallery (Edmonton, AB) and the University of the Arts, Philadelphia (USA). She has also shown in group exhibitions at the International Print Center (USA) and the 2nd Grand River International Printmaking Exhibition (China). She has participated in residencies at Open Studio in Toronto, Ontario and St. Michael's Printshop in St. John's, Newfoundland. (www.jillhoyou.com)

Heather Huston is assistant professor at the Alberta University of the Arts. She has exhibited widely in group exhibitions including *Kyoto Hanga, Printing Marks and Codes* (China), and *Di CARTA/PAPERMADE* (Italy). Recent solo exhibitions in Canada include *The Body, Stranger* at the Vernon Public Art Gallery in British Columbia; and *Shift* at SNAP Gallery in Edmonton, Alberta. Huston's work is in the collection of over 15 major institutions, including Crvena Komuna (Montenegró); Purdue University Galleries (USA); and City of Burnaby, Permanent Art Collection (Canada). (www.hhuston.com)

Bernie Krewski has lived with the impact of throat cancer, including facial disfigurement and various forms of interdisciplinary reconstruction, for 14 years. When he lost his natural speaking voice for nearly a year, he gained unique insights into human behaviour. His previous career in health care, especially mental health, was interwoven with an appreciation of the arts. While a dance metaphor poignantly symbolizes many aspects of his recovery, it also represents a sense of meaningful celebration and ecstasy—recognizing the synthesis of the ground-breaking achievements of sound medical practice and innovation with trendsetting artistic expression. Feeling distinctively human is the result.

Lianne McTavish is professor in the Department of Art & Design at the University of Alberta. Her research on early modern French visual culture, the history of the body, and critical museum theory has been funded by the Social Sciences and Humanities Research Council of Canada, the Hannah Institute for the History of Medicine, and the Killam Trust. In addition to numerous articles, she has published three monographs, including *Defining the Modern Museum* (2013). She is also completing two more books, one of which centres on small town and rural museums in Alberta (albertamuseumsproject.com). McTavish regularly curates exhibitions of contemporary art.

Suresh Nayar is a maxillofacial prosthodontist at the Institute for Reconstructive Sciences in Medicine and associate professor in the Division of Otolaryngology in the Department of Surgery, University of Alberta. Nayar's clinical work includes oral rehabilitation of head and neck cancer and craniofacial trauma patients. His research work focuses on patient-reported outcome measures and improving quality of life in head and neck cancer patients, as well as methods to reduce the adverse effects of radiation therapy on oral function. He chairs the Oral and Dental Care Clinical Guideline Review Committee for Alberta Health Services' Provincial Head and Neck Tumour Team.

Bradley Necyk is a multimedia artist whose practice engages challenging questions and issues within medicine, such as mental health, pharmaceutics, experience of vulnerable populations, and biopolitics. Following a successful residency with Alberta Health Service's Transplant Services (2015–2016), he has been a visiting artist-researcher at the Centre for Addiction and Mental Health in Toronto, Ontario. He is currently completing doctoral research in the Department of Psychiatry using arts-based research-creation and auto-ethnographic approaches. He is also an instructor in the Department of Art & Design and Faculty of Pharmacy and Pharmaceutical Sciences at the University of Alberta. (www.bradnecyk.com)

Leslie O'Connor-Parsons was diagnosed with tongue cancer in 2014. Her treatment has involved surgery, radiation, and chemotherapy. She joined the "see me, hear me, heal me" project as a patient partner in 2015, and in 2016 she participated with health care providers and researchers in an Alberta-based head and neck cancer research priority setting project. In 2003, she completed a fine arts diploma at the Ontario College of Art and Design (now OCAD University). She currently lives and heals in Edmonton, Alberta.

Kyle Terrence is an emerging artist and filmmaker from the industrial heart of Alberta, Canada. He holds a Master of Fine Arts degree from the University of Alberta, where he developed his thesis, *Pilgrimage: Being in the End Times* (2016). His most recent work, *Embeddings* (2017), was exhibited at the People's Lodge (Edmonton, AB), where Terrence completed an Art & Design Graduate Student Association alumni-sponsored artist residency. Terrence works primarily in film, performance, sculpture, and photography. His work often thinks through various discourses including the sublime, ecology, eschatology, and theology. Terrence is currently an art instructor at MacEwan University and the University of Alberta. (www.kyleterrence.com)

Helen Vallianatos is an associate professor in the Department of Anthropology at the University of Alberta. Her research and teaching explore connections between food, gender, body, health, and identity, using both visual and qualitative methods. She has studied the food consumption of pregnant women in New Delhi, India. Her work has also explored changes in food and health practices among immigrants to Canada and how this is linked to gender and ethnocultural identities, as well as intergenerational negotiations within families related to food and health behaviours.

Minn N. Yoon, associate professor in the School of Dentistry at the University of Alberta, initiated the "see me, hear me, heal me" project. Her research focuses on improving oral health and care of under-served populations. Much of her research is qualitative in nature, and almost always involves a collaborative team that includes a wide range of partners, which has contributed to the growth and vitality of her research program. She continues to apply the initial "see me, hear me, heal me" framework in various projects as part of a larger Living Stories initiative (www.livingstories.ca), as she remains boldly aimed at changing the world.